The 30-Minute Fitness Solution

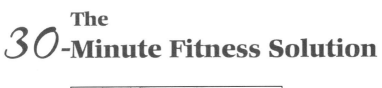

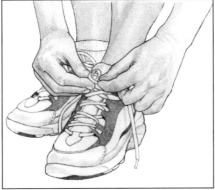

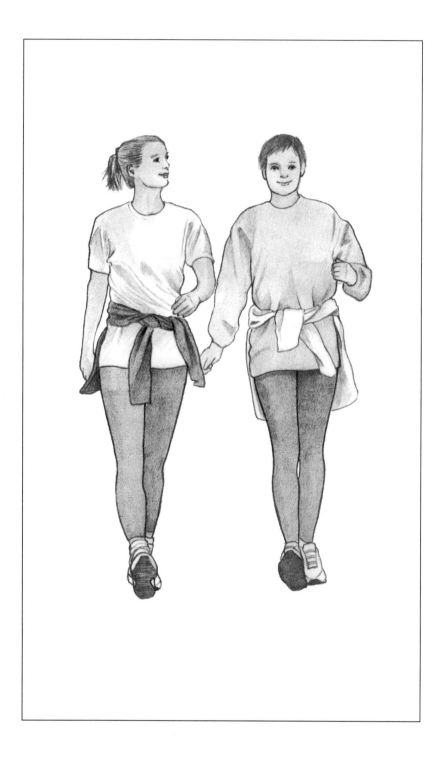

JoAnn Manson, M.D.
and Patricia Amend, M.A.

The *30*-Minute Fitness Solution

A Four-Step Plan
for Women of All Ages

Harvard University Press

Cambridge, Massachusetts, and London, England · 2001

Ilustrations by Susan Keller

This book is meant to educate, but it should not be used as a substitute for personal medical advice. The reader should consult her clinician for specific information concerning her individual medical condition. The authors have done their best to ensure that the information presented here is accurate up to the time of publication. However, as research and development are ongoing, it is possible that new findings may supersede some of the data presented here.

The authors, specialists, and publisher specifically disclaim any responsibility for any liability, loss, or risk, personal or otherwise, which is incurred as a consequence, directly or indirectly, of the use and application of any of the content of this book.

In cases where women are referred to by first name only, those names have been changed to preserve the privacy of interviewees.

Library of Congress Cataloging-in-Publication Data

Manson, JoAnn E.
    The 30-minute fitness solution : a four-step plan for women of all ages / JoAnn Manson and Patricia Amend.
        p.   cm.
    Includes bibliographical references and index.
    ISBN 0-674-00479-5
        1. Fitness walking.   2. Physical fitness for women.
    3. Walking—Health aspects.   4. Women—Health and hygiene.
    I. Title: Thirty minute fitness solution.   II. Amend, Patricia.
    III. Title.

RA781.65 .M36   2001
613.7'045—dc21   00-047185

Preface

Despite all the technological advances in modern medicine, physical activity is as close as we've come to a "magic bullet" for improving health. This doesn't have to mean long, sweaty workouts in the gym or five-mile runs before dawn. In fact, that tired old adage "No pain, no gain" is yesterday's medicine. Over the past few years, researchers have gathered compelling and very consistent evidence that moderate physical activity—something as simple as a brisk walk every day—can help you live healthier and live longer. Sadly, many women don't know this. Equally alarming, those who have heard about the benefits of moderate activity often find it difficult to squeeze some exercise into days already crammed with too many other must-do's. This book, which draws from my experiences as a clinician, medical researcher, wife, and mother, is intended to help make an active life-style a reality for women of all ages and circumstances.

The seeds for this book were planted more than 15 years ago when I was a medical resident and then an endocrinology fellow in Boston. Each week I saw dozens of patients with diabetes, high blood pressure, high cholesterol, heart disease, and many other chronic health problems. Treating these conditions can be difficult, and there is no guarantee that treatment will check the disease or its complications. It was common knowledge at the time that exercise could help control many of these conditions, and there were some early hints that it might even prevent them in the first place. I became fascinated by the potential role of exercise as a "health elixir" and have been following that idea ever since, through my work for a doctorate in public health at the Harvard School of Public Health and later as a medical researcher with the Nurses' Health Study, the Women's Health Initiative, and other large-scale studies of women.

This book grew out of a 1996 editorial in the *New England Journal of Medicine* that I wrote with a colleague at Harvard Medical School and the Harvard School of Public Health, Dr. I-Min Lee. Entitled "Exercise for Women—How Much Pain for Optimal Gain?" the editorial pointed out that for some women, prolonged, high-intensity exercise may have hazards as well as benefits. For some women, the hazards include irregular menstrual periods or a complete cessation of menstruation (amenorrhea), hormonal changes that can cause infertility and osteoporosis, and common injuries such as sprains and tendinitis. Given these very real risks, our editorial raised the question: How much exercise do women really need to protect their health?

The answer comes from a large body of evidence that highlights the health benefits of moderate-intensity exercise, including activities as simple as brisk walking. Together with my colleagues in the Nurses' Health Study, we have found that such activity is linked to a lower risk of heart disease, stroke, type 2 (adult-onset) diabetes, certain kinds of cancer, and other chronic diseases in women. Many other studies have shown similar benefits in women and men.

I know that merely telling my patients about the benefits of exercise or encouraging them to do it isn't enough, even when I write out an "exercise prescription" to walk 30 minutes a day. They hear the message but, heartbreakingly, few are able to follow through on a long-term basis. I don't blame them one bit, because I know the barriers they face. As a wife, mother, clinician, researcher, and chief of a busy research division at Brigham and Women's Hospital in Boston, I can identify with the feeling that adding one more thing, even something as simple and enjoyable as a daily walk, is out of the question. Finding time for exercise is something I have struggled with throughout my adult life. I've made it a priority, though, because I came to realize that the best thing I can do for my family is to stay healthy for as long as I can.

A major goal of this book is to make sure that women know that regular exercise is one of the best things they can do to prevent heart disease, stroke, diabetes, osteoporosis, some cancers, and other chronic diseases. That exercise is the absolute foundation for any *successful* weight-loss program. And that it can reduce stress, improve mood, make you feel better about your body, and give you a new outlook on life. It's true. Moderate exercise can do all of these things.

But the question remains, how do you get started? How do you change your habit of being inactive to active? What do you do, day to day?

Because I wanted this book to be practical as well as informative, I asked Patricia Amend, an extraordinarily talented journalist and health communicator, to join me as co-author. Pat has dealt with the same kinds of issues I have throughout her life and has written articles targeted toward fitness professionals for the last 15 years.

We devised a four-step approach to making exercise a pleasant, daily habit, drawing on several years of Pat's work with the noted sports psychologist Dr. James Annesi. Those steps are:

- **Plan:** set a goal, say, fitting into that mother-of-the-bride dress, and decide how to reach it
- **Proceed:** get up and get out, and put that plan into practice
- **Record:** keep track of your exercise and how it makes you feel while monitoring your progress
- **Reward:** choose small treats that keep you motivated and acknowledge the worthwhile effort that you've made

Together, Pat and I worked very hard to present the research on the health benefits of exercise in an easy-to-read, easy-to-digest manner. We have also detailed a number of ways to add 30 minutes of activity into even the busiest of days—which include several stretching and strength-training routines that will help keep you limber and strong. Make use of these, and you'll be in better shape to enjoy your life while preventing osteoporosis and broken bones, as well as other chronic diseases.

If exercise isn't already part of your lifestyle, I urge you to add 30 minutes of activity to your daily routine. This small but radical change will improve your health and your mood and revitalize your life. I hope that *The 30-Minute Fitness Solution* gives you the tools you need to make this change for yourself—and for those who love you.

JoAnn Manson, M.D.
Brigham and Women's Hospital
Harvard Medical School
Boston, Massachusetts

Contents

Boxes

This book is dedicated to our families

The
30-Minute Fitness Solution

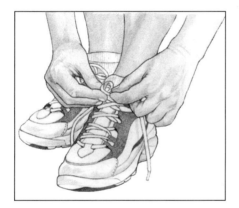

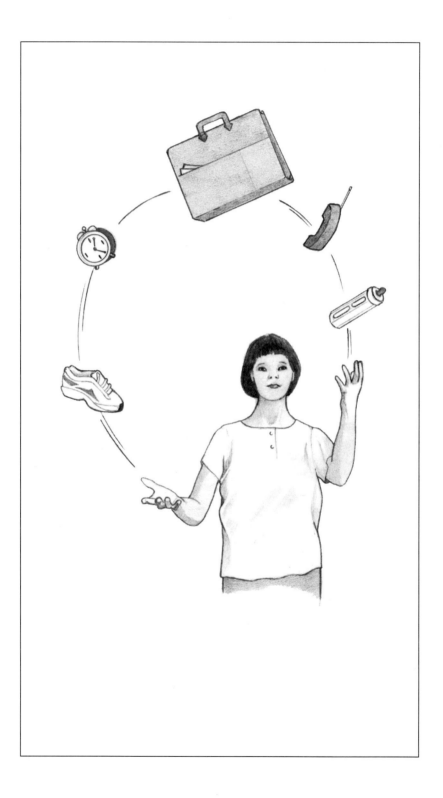

"I thought I could change the world. It took me a hundred
years to figure out I can't change the world. I can only
change Bessie. And honey, that ain't easy either."

    Annie Elizabeth "Bessie" Delany (1891–1995), African-American
    dentist, autobiographer, and centenarian

Introduction

Have you been promising yourself that you're going to start getting
some exercise? For many of us, this is a ritual resolution we make on
New Year's Day, or a birthday, or when we're feeling down or old or
overweight. We all have our reasons—to lose those extra pounds that
appeared from who knows where, to firm up that soft post-pregnancy
belly, to regain the energy we had ten years ago, to *not* have a heart
attack like a cousin did at age 59 or end up hunched over from osteoporosis like our mothers.

What's stopping you? Probably that four-letter word that few of us
can ever get enough of—TIME. Juggling family and work every day
is hard enough; tossing in a third obligation—to get some exercise—
may seem like an impossible feat. But it doesn't have to be.

Part of the problem may be your perception of exercise. There was
a time when the slogan "No pain, no gain" ruled the fitness world.
The leading health organizations said we needed long stretches of
vigorous activity several times a week—miles and miles of jogging,
swimming, hiking, and biking, or hours and hours of tennis and aerobics. Less than that, they told us, just wouldn't do much good. What's
more, the concept of "vigorous activity"—roughly translated as
sweaty activity—isn't appealing to many women.

That prescription of extended, huffing-and-puffing exertion is yesterday's medicine. Based on several long-term studies of physical activity and health, including Harvard's Nurses' Health Study (a land-

1

mark study that you'll hear a lot about in these chapters), today's recommendations call for 30 minutes of *moderate* activity—something like brisk walking—on most days of the week. Even better, those 30 minutes can be broken up into easier-to-schedule segments of 10 or 15 minutes each. For optimal health, the recommendations suggest two short strength-training sessions, and most experts also suggest some daily stretching exercises to keep you flexible—all of this amounting to less than an hour a week.

This simple prescription for maintaining or improving your health is really wonderful news for any woman who can walk and lift light weights. Most of us can find 30 minutes somewhere in our days for a brisk walk. Not only is brisk walking more practical and easier than vigorous activity for most women, it is just as effective and may also be safer. For some women, prolonged, high-intensity exercise may have hazards as well as benefits, ranging from irregular menstrual periods to infertility to osteoporosis (all caused by the hormonal changes brought about by intense exercise), as well as common injuries such as sprains and tendinitis.

Given that vigorous activity has risks as well as benefits, how much exercise do women really need to protect their health? A good answer comes from the Nurses' Health Study (NHS), which was started in 1976 at Harvard's Brigham and Women's Hospital to examine the health effects of various contraceptive practices among women. Since then, it has evolved into an exceptionally fruitful investigation of the roles played by diet, exercise, and other lifestyle factors in the prevention of heart conditions, cancer, diabetes, and other diseases. In 1986 investigators in this study asked more than 72,000 healthy female nurses detailed questions about their physical activity, and then asked them again in 1988 and 1992. Eight years after the first questionnaire, the women were divided into five groups based on average amount of physical activity. Substantially fewer of the nurses who walked briskly for about three hours a week (or its equivalent) outside of work had a heart attack or died from heart disease during the study period than did the nurses who were essentially inactive. More vigorous activity, such as running or aerobic dance, was associated with only slightly greater reductions in heart disease risk than brisk walking. Equally encouraging, even those women who became active in middle age or later were less likely to have a heart attack or die from heart disease than their counterparts who remained inactive. Similar benefits from walking and other moderate-intensity activities were found for type 2 (adult-onset) diabetes, stroke, and several other chronic diseases.

As the NHS and other studies have shown, vigorous activity is perfectly fine for some women. It provides some degree of additional protection against disease, mostly heart disease, over and above moderate activity. Vigorous sports activities can also inspire a high level of confidence and a sense of accomplishment that benefit women throughout their lives. We certainly encourage women with athletic ability and interest to pursue the sports they enjoy. For the rest of us, though, moderate activity is good enough to protect our health.

Moderate activity pays off in many ways. New research shows that 30 minutes of brisk walking or other equally energetic activity on a regular basis can:

- Reduce your risk of dying prematurely
- Help protect you from a long list of chronic, potentially disabling diseases, including heart disease, high blood pressure, stroke, diabetes, osteoporosis, and some kinds of cancer
- Help control your weight
- Strengthen your muscles and thus decrease the threat of falling and breaking a hip or other bone
- Improve your mood and reduce stress
- Help you feel better and look better

These benefits and others are detailed in the Surgeon General's landmark report on *Physical Activity and Health,* which we will describe in more detail later.

A Practical Plan

Simply knowing the hazards of inactivity and the multiple benefits of exercise isn't enough incentive to get most of us on our feet. What we need is help carving out time during the day to exercise and a plan for sticking with it. That's why we have written this book. We have devised different routines that you can work into almost any kind of day. We have also put together a variety of strategies that will encourage you to think about physical activity in a whole new light, and a series of questionnaires that will help you plot out a workable plan, record your progress, and stay focused on your goals.

What we've compiled between these covers will be relevant to you whether you are 25 or 75; whether you've never had children, are pregnant now, have children at home, or have grown children with independent lives; whether you are years from menopause, are going through menopause now, or passed through it many years ago; whether you are currently healthy or are living with a disease or other medical condition. Physical activity is important to every woman, through every stage of our lives, for as long as we live.

As busy women ourselves, we are all too familiar with the barriers that prevent women from starting and sticking with an exercise program. Both of us have, at one time or another, planned to become more active without doing much about it, or started exercising only to lapse a few weeks later. And we've heard endless variations on these themes over the years from other women. So our single aim for this book is to create exercise programs that are practical for a variety of women—single working women, stay-at-home mothers, women who race between child care and a full-time job, as well as older women who may have a bit more free time.

In the pages that follow, we discuss why you need exercise to stay healthy through every stage of your life, how to go about building an exercise habit, what to do about exercise if you already have a medical condition, and ways you can help those you love become more active. We also suggest some simple changes in your diet that will further boost the benefits of physical activity.

Our goals are down-to-earth. We want to help you discover that physical activity improves not just your long-term health but also your day-to-day mental outlook, adding a level of richness and satisfaction to your life that you may not have imagined was possible with such small, simple adjustments. We also want to help you translate the vague notion "I need to exercise" into action. Through this book we *work with you* to help you schedule 30 minutes of moderate activity into your day, along with 15 to 20 minutes of strength training twice a week.

We begin by describing the key research that shows how physical activity helps ward off disease (Chapters 1 and 2). Next, we lay out a four-step plan for creating an exercise habit (Chapter 3). It consists of planning your active lifestyle (Chapter 4), proceeding with exercise, both moderate activity and strength training (Chapter 5), recording your progress (Chapter 6), and rewarding your effort (Chapter 7). In Chapter 8 we offer three detailed strength-training programs to help you get started with this small but very important piece of your exercise plan. In Chapter 9 we provide tips for buying home exercise equipment, as well as four beginners' programs so that you'll make good use of the machine once you get it home. For those who prefer to train in a health or sports club, we also offer advice on how to choose a club that suits your particular needs.

A healthy diet (see Chapter 10) maximizes the benefits of physical activity. After helping you evaluate your current eating habits, we invite you to explore your thoughts about your body and how they affect, and are affected by, diet and exercise. In Chapter 11 we describe in detail the many scientific studies that bolster our confidence in the program we describe in this book. If you already have a medical condition, be sure to read Chapter 12, where we review the latest research on the benefits of physical activity for people with heart disease, high blood pressure, high cholesterol, stroke, obesity, diabetes, osteoporosis, arthritis, and cancer. We also recommend specific activities for people with these conditions.

Because exercise can have a dramatic effect on one's mental and emotional outlook, and because women are twice as likely to suffer from depression as men, in Chapter 13 we explore the latest research on the psychological benefits of physical activity. And in Chapter 14, we look at physical activity across the stages of a woman's life—before pregnancy, during pregnancy, after a baby arrives, during middle adulthood, during menopause, and into old age. We pay special attention to the importance of strength training for mobility and independent living in later life. Finally, because physical activity is important to everyone, we devote Chapter 15 to ways you can help others close to you add moderate levels of activity to their daily routine.

Thirty minutes of moderate daily exercise can lead to improved health and greater happiness. We urge you to try it—and make this life-changing and life-saving discovery for yourself!

1

The Best Investment You'll Ever Make

"I have tried several times to be more active but always seem to end up back where I started—doing very little," says 51-year-old Marilyn. "I see women out walking in my neighborhood early in the morning, or circling the pond in the evening, and I'd really like to join them. But in the morning I barely have enough time to get myself out the door—let alone my two teenagers—and the end of the day, after work, is even worse. Just when I'd like to unwind with a walk or something, I'm either back in the car to pick up my daughter or son from soccer practice or hurrying to make dinner. Weekends I'm pooped, but that's the only time for housework and all the other things left over from the rest of the week."

Sound familiar? At first glance, it looks as though Marilyn is stuck until her children leave home for college or she quits her job. Actually, Marilyn figured out a simpler solution. By hopping off the subway two stops early, she now squeezes in a 15-minute walk to work without significantly lengthening her commute. Walking back to the same station in the evening adds another 15 minutes. Voilá! 30 minutes of exercise in a normal workday.

"It took a while to get used to, and I would sometimes find excuses to stay on the train," Marilyn admits. "Now I look forward to the walk. Partly because I know I'm doing something good for myself. And partly because I like to look at all the people downtown. I try to figure out which ones are doing the same thing I am—exercising on

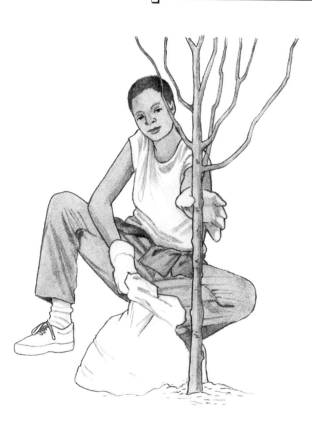

the way to work—and which ones are just hurrying. Plus I met a neighbor who works in the next building, and she and I schedule in a little 'walk and talk' twice a week."

Exercise was a hard sell for Marilyn. It took a week of chest pain, several days of tests, a lot of anxiety, and a less-than-rosy prediction about the state of her heart to get Marilyn to start an exercise program. We hope you won't wait for similar bad news about yourself or someone close to you before you convert your promises into action. Unfortunately, too many women (and men) do just that. Here are a few sobering statistics:

- Heart disease, stroke, cancer, and diabetes cause 80% of all illness, disability, and death among women in the United States, and each of these conditions is associated with inactivity. The combination of inactivity and poor diet accounts for 22% to 40% of deaths due to heart disease or stroke, 30% of deaths due to diabetes, and 20% to 60% of deaths due to cancer.

- More than one third of all women in the United States between the ages of 18 and 64 and nearly half of those over age 65 do not exercise at all. Less than half of all women exercise three times a week. African-American women, Hispanic women, and Asian women are less likely to exercise than white women. Across all age groups, women get less exercise than men.

- The top five sources of calories in the average American diet are bread (9.8%); beef (7.0%); milk (5.7%); cakes, cookies, quick breads, and donuts (5.5%); and soft drinks (4.1%). Also in the top 10 are salad dressings, mayonnaise, and margarine. There's not a vegetable in sight until white potatoes at number 12.

- This combination of inactivity and poor diet is fattening us up. An astounding 54% of Americans are considered overweight, and one third qualify for the medical diagnosis of obesity, which means weighing at least 20% more than is recommended for one's height. That adds up to about 32 million American women and 26 million men who are considered obese—a bad sign for the present and the future, given that excess weight increases the chances of developing heart disease, diabetes, and some cancers.

If you think about it for a moment, both a sedentary lifestyle and a poor diet stem from many small choices people make every day. Do I have a donut for breakfast or some cereal with skim milk? A burger and fries for lunch or a turkey sandwich and a salad? Do I plop down and watch television after dinner or take a brisk walk around the neighborhood? These small choices add up, sometimes with deadly results. We are finally coming to realize that sitting too much and eating the wrong foods are just as lethal as smoking, with at least 300,000 deaths each year caused by the combination of inactivity and poor diet.

A Landmark: The 1996 Surgeon General's Report

Just as the 1964 Surgeon General's report on *Smoking and Health* opened our eyes to the dangers of cigarettes, the 1996 Surgeon General's report on *Physical Activity and Health* revealed the strength of the link between a sedentary lifestyle and chronic disease, and between physical activity and good health. As is so often the case in science, information on the connection between activity and health emerged gradually, a study here, a study there, a conference here, a book chapter there. The major contribution of the Surgeon General's report was to pull all of this information together. This exhaustive 278-page document reviewed decades of research from many disciplines on the connections between lifestyle choices and disease and concluded that lack of exercise was clearly related to the epidemic rates of heart disease, stroke, cancer, and diabetes in this country.

But then the scientists who contributed to the report went one step further: they offered proof that regular, moderate physical activity can do more than help prevent these diseases—it can dramatically improve one's quality of life by reducing symptoms of depression, stress, and anxiety and by enhancing one's ability to meet the physical demands of daily life. The Surgeon General's report, produced by a coalition of the nation's leading health organizations, including the Centers for Disease Control and Prevention, the National Center for Chronic Disease Prevention and Health Promotion, and the President's Council on Physical Fitness and Sports, set the stage for today's new views on exercise.

The report pointed out that exercise need not be vigorous or difficult to be beneficial, and that a moderate amount of moderate-intensity exercise offers protection from many lifestyle-related diseases. The government's recommendations boiled down to these:

- Everyone should get at least 30 minutes of physical activity on most—preferably all—days of the week.
- Everyone should also do exercises or activities designed to strengthen muscles at least twice a week.

That's the minimum needed to reap the health benefits of physical activity. Of course, as the report points out, "Additional health benefits can be gained through greater amounts of physical activity. People who can maintain a regular regimen of activity that is of longer duration or of more vigorous intensity are likely to derive the greater benefit." In other words, if you can do more, more power—and more health benefits—to you. But doing more is not essential to achieving good health.

Women Have Special Activity Needs

Most women think that breast cancer is the number-one killer of women. That's just not true. Breast cancer is undeniably a terrible disease, killing more than 40,000 women a year, but heart disease, stroke, and other cardiovascular diseases kill more than 10 times that many—at least 500,000 women a year.* Prior to menopause, women are protected by estrogen and other factors and so tend to develop heart disease roughly 10 years later than men. But once estrogen levels start dropping dramatically around menopause, heart disease in women increases, and within a decade or so it is running rampant. By age 65, women face almost the same risk of heart disease as men.

Regular physical activity can improve these odds, however, by reducing risk factors such as high cholesterol, high blood pressure, and high blood sugar, all of which increase one's chances of developing heart disease. Exercise has also been shown to prevent heart attacks and deaths due to heart disease. Here are some statistics suggesting why it is even more critical for women than men to make physical activity a top priority:

- While death from heart disease has been on the decline for both sexes since the 1960s, the decline is less pronounced in women. In general, men have made more substantial reductions in risk factors such as cholesterol and high blood pressure, perhaps because messages about risk reduction have been targeted more toward men.
- Women are less likely to survive heart attacks than men. Data from the Myocardial Infarction Triage and Intervention Registry reveal that 16% of women die in the hospital after a heart attack, compared with 11% of men. In addition, fewer women then men are

* In this book, we will use the term "heart disease" in place of the more specific labels of coronary heart disease or coronary artery disease that are generally used by physicians. In general, these two conditions refer to problems caused by narrowing and/or blockage of the coronary arteries—the arteries that provide oxygen and nourishment to the heart muscle.

likely to live through the first year after a severe heart attack. Women who undergo coronary artery bypass surgery to replace one or more clogged arteries in the heart have almost double the mortality rates of men, and more women than men need a second operation within five years of the first. Many of these problems may be related to the fact that women have smaller arteries than men, that they tend to develop heart disease later in life than men and hence may have complications from other diseases, and that women don't necessarily have the "classic" symptoms of a heart attack or other forms of heart disease that would alert them to seek help early on.

- After menopause, women have higher levels of cholesterol than do men of similar ages, and a larger proportion of women have high cholesterol, defined as a reading of 240 milligrams per deciliter or higher. According to the National Center for Health Statistics, about 27% of women aged 45 to 54 have high cholesterol, while 41% of those aged 55 to 74 have high cholesterol.
- Until age 55 or so, women are less likely than men to have high blood pressure. After that, though, the numbers reverse. Among people aged 55 to 64, 44% of women and 43% of men have high blood pressure. Those proportions rise to 61% for women and 57% for men between age 65 and 74, and 77% for women and 64% for men aged 75 and older.
- At almost every age, a higher proportion of women are overweight than men.
- While adult-onset (type 2) diabetes affects similar numbers of women and men, for some reason it has a greater impact on women's hearts. Rates of heart disease are 3 to 7 times higher in women with diabetes than in women without the disease, compared with 2 to 3 times higher in men with diabetes than in men without it.
- The situation is even worse for African-American, Hispanic, and Native American women. High blood pressure, type 2 diabetes, excess weight, and physical inactivity are more prevalent among these women than among white women.

Where Are You Now?

If you are reading this book, you're probably at a crossroads. Our guess is that you're tired of your own procrastination, and you'd like to do something about it now. The problem is, you're not quite sure what to do or how to get started. The first step is to answer the simple questionnaires in Boxes 1 and 2. They will reveal a lot about how you feel.

If these inventories show that you need or want to make some changes, what's holding you back? Maybe you've tried before but weren't successful, and you aren't sure where you went wrong. Let's look at it a different way. You probably didn't "go wrong." Getting

BOX 1

Lifestyle Inventory

1. **During a typical week day, do you walk or get any other kind of exercise?**
   Rarely   Almost always
   1 2 3 4 5 6 7 8 9 10

2. **What about on weekends?**
   Rarely   Almost always
   1 2 3 4 5 6 7 8 9 10

3. **Do you find yourself out of breath when doing routine tasks?**
   Rarely   Almost always
   1 2 3 4 5 6 7 8 9 10

4. **Do you get sore muscles after doing routine tasks?**
   Rarely   Almost always
   1 2 3 4 5 6 7 8 9 10

5. **Do you have a tendency to eat too much, or eat too many high-fat foods?**
   Rarely   Almost always
   1 2 3 4 5 6 7 8 9 10

Items 1 and 2 refer to activity level; items 3 and 4 to functional fitness; item 5 to diet.

BOX 2

Mood/Body Image Inventory

1. Do you feel sad, discouraged, or low?
Rarely   Almost always
1 2 3 4 5 6 7 8 9 10

2. Do you feel tired or sluggish?
Rarely   Almost always
1 2 3 4 5 6 7 8 9 10

3. Do you feel tense, anxious, or uneasy?
Rarely   Almost always
1 2 3 4 5 6 7 8 9 10

4. Do you feel energetic and full of pep?
Rarely   Almost always
1 2 3 4 5 6 7 8 9 10

5. On a scale of 1 to 4, with 1 as the lowest level of satisfaction, check the box in each row that best describes how you feel about your:

Face	1	2	3	4
Lower torso	1	2	3	4
Mid torso	1	2	3	4
Upper torso	1	2	3	4
Weight	1	2	3	4
Overall appearance	1	2	3	4

Item 1 refers to feelings of depression; item 2 to feelings of fatigue; item 3 to feelings of stress or anxiety; item 4 to energy level; item 5 to body image.

Sources: Adapted from D. M. McNair, M. Lorr, and I. F. Droppelman, *Manual for the Profile of Mood States* (San Diego: Educational and Industrial Testing Service, 1992); T. F. Cash, *The Multidimensional Body-Self Relations Questionnaire Users' Manual* (unpub.ms., Old Dominion University); T. A. Brown, T. F. Cash, and T. J. Mikula, "Additional Body Image Assessment: Factor Analysis of the Body-Self Relations Questionnaire," *Journal of Personality Assessment* 55 (1990): 135–144.

rid of a bad habit like inactivity, or adding a new *anything* to your life, is a much harder task than most of us admit. Each day we reinforce the patterns of our lives, and breaking these patterns takes more than just deciding to do it. It usually requires a carefully constructed plan, one that begins with small and realistic changes, like walking out the front door and taking a short walk for 10 minutes.

There are plenty of psychological barriers to becoming more active. Many of us grew up at a time when exercise was considered unfeminine, or just for athletes or tomboys. It's also common for women to feel that our responsibilities to our families and jobs come first, and exercise comes second, or third, or dead last. Some women also feel so ill at ease with their bodies that they can't bring themselves to exercise in public.

You can get past these roadblocks. No need to leap them or hurdle them, just put one foot in front of the other and walk around them. We hope this book will encourage you to join the ranks of women who are doing just that—literally one step at a time. We will guide you toward making small changes in your activity and diet that will, over time, lead to a healthier, happier, more productive life. We'd like to show you that *doing something* is entirely possible, especially when you have a workable plan.

Small Changes Can Make a Difference

If you recognize yourself in the somewhat scary statistics above, or have simply known for a long time that you need to make a change, keep in mind that it need not be a momentous, revolutionary, 180° turnabout. You can start with one or two very small changes, say taking a 10-minute walk at lunchtime and trading in butter for jam on your morning toast. Once these changes are part of your routine, you can expand a bit here, do a bit more there. Pretty soon, you've engineered yourself a newer, more healthy lifestyle. Once you discover the power of making small changes for yourself, we hope you'll use the influence you have as a partner, mother, sister, daughter, aunt, teacher, co-worker, or friend to help others make these important changes as well. In a small and personal way, you can help stop our nation's epidemic of lifestyle-related diseases.

Exercise: The Core of an Active Lifestyle

If it takes only 30 minutes of moderate activity a day to achieve better health, you may be wondering, "If I live a fairly active life, do I really need to exercise?" Say you're always running up and down the stairs chasing after your kids, or constantly carrying bags of groceries or heaping laundry baskets. Or you have a 9-to-5 job and you regularly take the stairs instead of the elevator, or walk several blocks to catch a bus or subway, or purposely park your car in the farthest spot available in the office parking lot so you'll have to walk the distance. Don't these things count?

Absolutely! And we urge you to continue doing these things; they are vital to good health. The ideal goal is being as physically active as possible throughout the day while also working in some activity that boosts your heart rate for at least 30 minutes—all at once, or spread out over two or three sessions. If you're like most women, this means getting your heart beating to between 60% and 80% of its maximum rate. (See Chapter 5 to calculate your maximum heart rate.) In this book, we will talk a lot about brisk walking for several reasons: it elevates your heart rate, it doesn't require any training or special equipment, it doesn't cost anything, and you can do it anywhere and in (almost) any weather.

Walking isn't everyone's cup of tea, though. There are plenty of alternatives. Biking, either outdoors or inside on a stationary bike; walking on a treadmill or stairclimber; swimming; dancing—you're limited only by your imagination and interests. Throughout the book, we'll refer to this main activity as your *core activity*—the one that gives your heart its daily charge.

Do It for Fun

There is another benefit of exercise beyond maintaining good health—it's a lot of fun. As the singer/actress Dinah Shore once put it, "I have never thought of participating in sports just for the sake of doing it for exercise or as a means to lose weight. And I've never taken up a sport just because it was a social fad. I really enjoy playing. It is a vital part of my life."

Some women relish the solitude they get from a morning walk or an after-work session on the treadmill. Others find that exercising with others offers an opportunity to catch up with old friends or even to make new ones. For still others, exercise opens unexpected doors.

"I've always been a walker," explains Sarah, who is 64 years old. "When my children were little, I used to walk every day with them in the stroller. These days, walking helps me avoid gaining weight. Three years ago, my husband and I did our first 10-kilometer Volkswalk, 'a walk of the people,' at a local park. It's an idea that came over from Germany. Since then, we've done over 300 walks. Most of our vacations now consist of walking. Last year we went to Wyoming and Arizona, and we hit other nearby states on those trips. It was gorgeous. The people who lay out these walks are locals, so they know the points of interest. They take you through beautiful wooded areas, parks, and try to give you the best of their area. Sometimes the new people we meet are as much fun as the walk itself."

The chapters that follow will include the stories of women like Marilyn and Sarah who have managed to become—and stay—active, often despite physical limitations or crammed schedules. They will share with you how they find time for physical activity, why they feel it's important to make the effort, and how being physically fit enhances their lives. As you meet these women, you'll discover that each one has come to the same conclusion: Creating an active lifestyle that includes regular exercise and a balanced diet is the best investment in yourself you'll ever make.

Points to Remember

- Four of the six top causes of death for women are associated with inactivity.
- After menopause, women develop heart disease, stroke, cancer, and diabetes at rates similar to those of men, but the outcome in women is often worse.
- A sedentary lifestyle is the result of many small choices you make every day. Becoming more active involves equally small choices.
- The 1996 landmark Surgeon General's report on *Physical Activity*

and Health recommends that everyone get 30 minutes of moderate activity on most days of the week, along with two strength-training sessions a week. Similar guidelines have been endorsed by the American Heart Association and several other leading health organizations.

- Pick an activity that resonates with your interests and history, then just start doing it!

"Think like a queen. A queen is not afraid to fail. Failure is
another steppingstone to greatness."

Oprah Winfrey (1954–), TV personality,
actress, producer

2

Exercise,
Nature's Medicine

How could something as simple as a brisk, 30-minute walk every day
and two sessions of strength training per week have such powerful effects on health as those we described in Chapter 1? To answer this
question, we'll start by discussing the health hazards of inactivity.
Then we'll move on to what we mean by *fitness* and show you how
your body adapts and becomes stronger with continued exercise.
We'll also describe some of the biological mechanisms by which moderate exercise improves health.

With this knowledge, you'll immediately see the value and power
of moderate activity. You'll also better understand why a balanced
program that consists of aerobic activity, strength training, and
stretching is essential to your health and well-being through all the
stages of your life.

The Hazards of Inactivity

We begin life as active creatures, kicking and twisting in the warm
waterworld of our mothers. At birth we squirm and flail our tiny
arms. Infants move instinctively, and it's almost impossible to stop a
toddler from scooting around the house or the block. Our muscles require activity, even just the normal push and pull of everyday life, to
keep them healthy. Bind a broken arm or leg in an inflexible cast for
two months and the unused muscle begins to waste away. And even

18

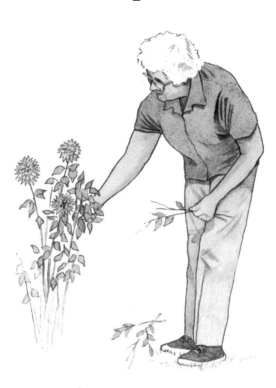

though you can't see them or flex them, hearts and lungs also need activity to keep from withering.

To examine the physiological and metabolic consequences of inactivity, researchers confined two groups of male volunteers to bed for up to three weeks. One group was made up of men whose normal life was sedentary, the other group of healthy young athletes. Despite this difference, both groups experienced profound declines in heart, lung, and circulatory system function within a matter of days; and the longer the period of inactivity, the greater the loss of function. Disturbances in metabolism were also seen within a few days of the start of bed rest, including early signs of type 2 (adult-onset) diabetes, loss of muscle protein, loss of bone mass, and a reduction in the amount of energy burned by the body at rest. Unfortunately, a similar but all-too-real scenario is played out every day in nursing homes, convalescence centers, and private residences around the world.

Clearly, the kind of relative inactivity (not exercising) that we're addressing in this book doesn't affect us as much as the absolute inactivity described in the experiment above. But it still takes its toll. Among women in the United States, the least active ones are the most likely to have a heart attack or stroke, develop adult-onset diabetes, be overweight, suffer from the bone-thinning condition known as osteoporosis, and face debilitating falls in old age.

Functional Fitness vs. Cardiorespiratory Fitness

When we use the word *fitness,* we mean functional fitness rather than cardiorespiratory fitness.

- **Functional fitness** is the ability to carry out the activities of everyday life without pain or discomfort, without shortness of breath, without your heart beating like crazy—in short, without limitation. Functional fitness comes from healthier and stronger lungs, heart, muscles, bones, and psyche.
- **Cardiorespiratory fitness** goes a step or two further and implies the kind of physical conditioning that you need for sustained, vigorous activity.

In other words, the 30 minutes of exercise that we suggest you do each day will protect you from lifestyle-related illnesses and allow you to perform daily tasks more easily. Along the way it will also improve how your heart, lungs, and muscles work, particularly if you have been relatively inactive up until now. But it will not give you the level of fitness you need to run a marathon, climb a mountain, or go cross-country skiing in rugged terrain. That will take a bit more effort. If you are interested in improving your cardiorespiratory fitness to the point where you can engage in these vigorous activities, then we recommend that you join a health club or YMCA whose fitness professionals can guide you through an appropriate exercise program.

Contrary to the old axiom "No pain, no gain," pain is not an essential ingredient in a fitness program, and it isn't particularly good for you, especially when you have been relatively inactive. Instead, the route to functional fitness begins with a durable, consistent, easy-to-do exercise habit that doesn't make you uncomfortable.

Don't get us wrong—we aren't suggesting that you avoid vigorous activity. Vigorous activity is fine if you're healthy and you do it in moderation. As the Surgeon General's report on *Physical Activity and Health* points out, there is a dose-response relationship with physical activity. That is, the more you exercise, the more benefits you will get from it—provided, of course, you don't take it to extremes. In the Nurses' Health Study, women who walked at a brisk pace (a minimum of 3 miles per hour) for just 1 hour per week cut their risk of heart disease by 30%, whereas those who walked 3 hours or more per week, as we recommend in this book, cut their risk by 40%. Furthermore, the women who usually walked at a brisk pace were about half as likely to develop heart disease as the women who usually walked at a more casual pace (see Box 3).

Guidelines for exercise and physical activity have evolved considerably over the past 20 years. Until recently, they all recommended vigorous activity as the route to better health. In the early 1990s, though, as research on the benefits of moderate activity came to light, recommendations began to shift. The truly groundbreaking change came in 1992, when the American Heart Association released a position paper that fingered inactivity as a major risk factor for coronary artery disease and at the same time recognized and highlighted the multiple benefits of moderate exercise. That same year, the Centers for Disease Control and Prevention and the American College of Sports Medicine issued the following joint statement: "Every U.S. adult should accumulate 30 minutes or more of moderate intensity physical activity on most, preferably all, days of the week." This was based on scientific evidence that short bouts of activity totaling at least 30 minutes provide significant health benefits. The same recommendation was made by the National Institutes of Health in 1995, and in the Surgeon General's report on *Physical Activity and Health* in 1996.

Today, the American Heart Association's current recommendation "for most healthy people" reads: "For health benefits to the heart, lungs and circulation, perform any vigorous activity for at least 30 minutes, 3–4 days each week at 50% to 75% of maximum heart rate. Moderate physical activity for 30 minutes on most days provides some benefits. Physical activity need not be strenuous to bring health benefits. What is important is to include activity as part of the regular routine."

If you have been sedentary and choose to begin a balanced program that includes moderate aerobic exercise plus strength-training and stretching exercises, in a matter of weeks you'll find you have greater aerobic capacity, meaning that you will find yourself increasingly able to climb an extra flight of stairs with grocery bags or an

BOX 3

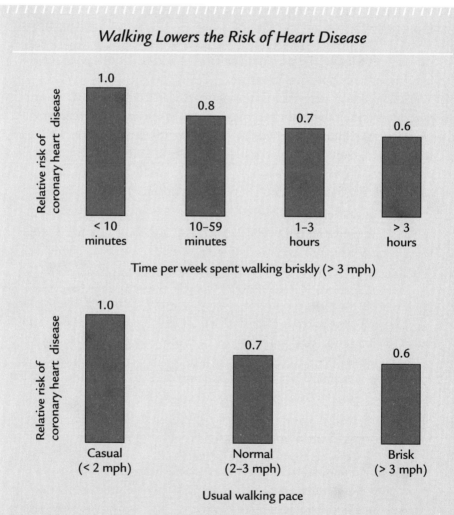

Walking Lowers the Risk of Heart Disease

Relative risk of coronary heart disease

1.0	0.8	0.7	0.6
< 10 minutes	10–59 minutes	1–3 hours	> 3 hours

Time per week spent walking briskly (> 3 mph)

Relative risk of coronary heart disease

1.0	0.7	0.6
Casual (< 2 mph)	Normal (2–3 mph)	Brisk (> 3 mph)

Usual walking pace

Source: Adapted from the Nurses' Health Study/Harvard's Brigham and Women's Hospital; *New England Journal of Medicine* 1999

armful of reports without becoming short of breath or feeling as though your heart is beating far too fast for comfort. You'll have the muscular strength, flexibility, and energy to fully enjoy recreational activities, whether you're hiking in the woods or playing volleyball at a picnic or dancing at a wedding. You'll do it with an ease of movement that you didn't have before—provided, of course, that you haven't pushed yourself beyond your physical limits. The good news is that those limits will continue to expand if you stick with your exercise program.

In other words, over time you will become more "fit." By this we mean you'll have the strength, endurance, and flexibility to be in control of your body and to enjoy optimum health and physical productivity. You'll sleep more deeply, handle stress better, and feel a greater sense of control over your life. You'll radiate a new sense of pride, power, and confidence—and peace of mind.

The Benefits of Weight-Bearing Aerobic Exercise

From a physiological standpoint, regular physical activity strengthens many systems in the body and ensures that important chemical processes vital to health keep functioning as they should. Women who are physically active are likely to have higher levels of the protective form of cholesterol and lower blood pressure, which translates into a reduced risk of having a heart attack or stroke (see Box 4). They are more likely to keep their body weight stable and have less body fat overall and in the abdominal area, which decreases their chances of developing type 2 (adult-onset) diabetes (see Box 5). They are also less likely to develop osteoporosis and certain types of cancers, including breast and colon cancers (see Box 6).

In short, weight-bearing aerobic exercise, which uses the major muscle groups of the body, helps you:

- Build a stronger, more efficient heart and lungs
- Maintain bone mass
- Stay strong and flexible
- Improve the ability of muscles and other tissues to use insulin
- Reduce and redistribute body fat
- Prevent certain forms of cancer

- Improve emotional well-being
- Lessen the effects of aging

Perhaps most important of all, women who were active at least 4 hours a week were 30% less likely to die during a 16-year period of the Nurses' Health Study. In other words, being active lowers the risk of mortality and early death (see Box 7).

BUILD A STRONGER, MORE EFFICIENT HEART AND LUNGS

The heart, blood vessels, and lungs deliver oxygen and nutrients to the body, rid it of carbon dioxide and waste products generated by cells, maintain body temperature and acid-base balance, and transport hormones from the endocrine glands to the appropriate organs. Aerobic activities are those that make the muscles, including the heart, demand more oxygen.

When you walk briskly or climb stairs, your muscles work harder

BOX 4

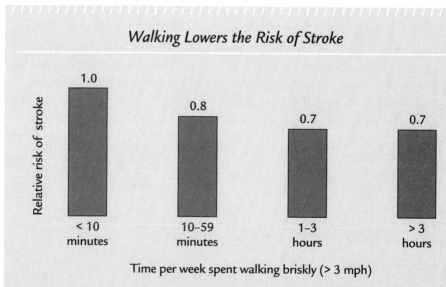

Walking Lowers the Risk of Stroke

Relative risk of stroke

1.0 — < 10 minutes
0.8 — 10–59 minutes
0.7 — 1–3 hours
0.7 — > 3 hours

Time per week spent walking briskly (> 3 mph)

Source: Adapted from the Nurses' Health Study/Harvard's Brigham and Women's Hospital; *JAMA* 2000

than usual. This sets off a physiological and chemical chain of events that rather quickly starts your heart beating faster and makes your breathing faster and deeper, a dual process aimed at bringing extra oxygen and energy to your muscles and removing the additional waste. As you continue walking or climbing, you may eventually have to stop. This is the point at which your cardiovascular and respiratory systems have reached their maximum and can no longer deliver the oxygen your muscles need to continue the activity. As an exercise physiologist would explain it, you've reached your maximum oxygen uptake, or VO_2 max.

The more you work the large muscle groups of your body, such as the arms or legs, the faster and harder your heart must beat to supply them with oxygen and energy. Regular exercise helps your cardiovascular and respiratory systems become more efficient at delivering oxygen and nutrients and removing wastes, allowing you to walk, climb stairs, or chase after your kids without becoming winded or fatigued. This *training effect* occurs because of an increase in cardiac output—

BOX 5

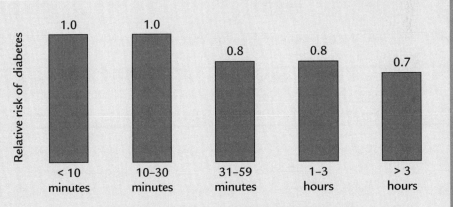

Walking Lowers the Risk of Type 2 (Adult-Onset) Diabetes

Relative risk of diabetes

| < 10 minutes | 10–30 minutes | 31–59 minutes | 1–3 hours | > 3 hours |
| 1.0 | 1.0 | 0.8 | 0.8 | 0.7 |

Time per week spent walking briskly (> 3 mph)

Source: Adapted from the Nurses' Health Study/Harvard's Brigham and Women's Hospital; *JAMA* 1999

BOX 6

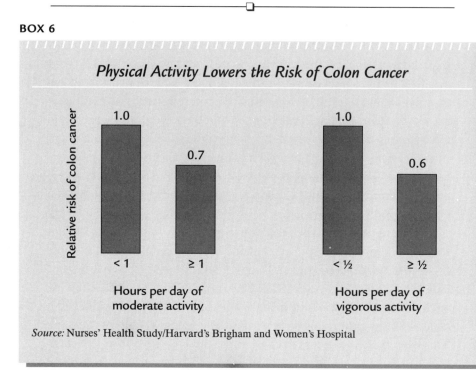

Physical Activity Lowers the Risk of Colon Cancer

Source: Nurses' Health Study/Harvard's Brigham and Women's Hospital

that is, the left ventricle of the heart pumps a greater volume of blood each minute, delivering more oxygen with less effort throughout the body.

As your heart becomes more efficient at pumping blood, it begins beating less often when you aren't active, lowering what is known as your *resting heart rate*. Your muscles also become more efficient at extracting oxygen from the blood as it passes through the intricate lattice of tiny blood vessels called capillaries. At the same time, exercise improves pulmonary ventilation—the ability of your lungs and blood vessels to flush your blood with oxygen and deliver that oxygen to the muscles and other tissues that need it. Training your lungs and blood vessels to deliver more oxygen per minute of activity lowers your blood pressure and improves your circulation.

Regular physical activity also increases blood levels of high-density lipoproteins (HDL, the "good" cholesterol), reduces blood levels of low-density lipoproteins (LDL, the "bad" cholesterol), and speeds up the clearance of triglycerides (another type of fat particle) from the bloodstream after a meal. In addition, it increases the muscles' ability to use insulin, which helps keep blood sugar levels relatively steady. All of these reduce the risk of both heart disease and adult-onset diabetes.

MAINTAIN BONE MASS

Bone isn't the hard and lifeless material you might think it is. Instead, it is living tissue that is constantly remodeled by the body. And like other tissues, bone is affected by diet and exercise.

Most healthy women build and store bone fairly efficiently until age 35 or so, if they get enough calcium in their diets. Around age 35 the scale tips, and bone loss begins to outpace bone building unless something is done to stop it. This process accelerates during menopause, when estrogen levels drop, and continues after menopause. If a women does nothing to shore up her infrastructure, she may develop osteoporosis, a condition in which bones become so porous that they compress or break easily. The bent-over posture and hip

BOX 7

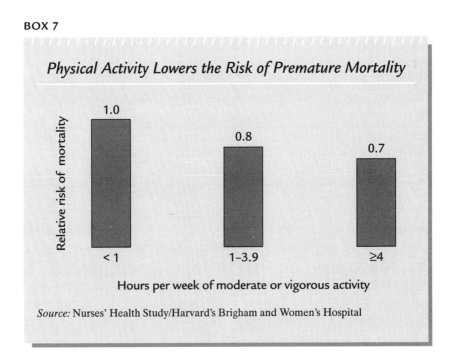

Physical Activity Lowers the Risk of Premature Mortality

Relative risk of mortality

1.0 — < 1
0.8 — 1–3.9
0.7 — ≥4

Hours per week of moderate or vigorous activity

Source: Nurses' Health Study/Harvard's Brigham and Women's Hospital

and wrist fractures that older women suffer are the most obvious signs of this disease.

Weight-bearing exercises—those that put an appropriate, healthy amount of mechanical stress on the bones—stimulate bone growth and help bones maintain their strength and density as women age. Walking, jogging, running, rope skipping, stair climbing, cross-country skiing, and rowing are all weight-bearing aerobic exercises because they work the arms, the legs, or both. (Swimming is not a weight-bearing exercise because the body is buoyed by the water; nor is cycling, because the body is supported by the bicycle.)

STAY STRONG AND FLEXIBLE

Without weight-bearing exercise, a woman loses approximately a half pound of muscle a year beginning at age 30 or so and continuing for the next 25 to 30 years. Men lose even more. There's usually no weight loss, though, because this lost muscle is replaced with fat. As the ratio of muscle mass to fat mass shrinks, the body burns fewer calories at rest and when active. In other words, the metabolic rate slows down. Weight gain usually follows, and this new weight is more fat, not more muscle. This is the phenomenon known not-so-affectionately as "middle-age spread." Strength training twice a week can help you keep the muscle you have which, in turn, can help you control your weight and maintain a healthy muscle-to-fat ratio. Two brief stretching sessions morning and night can also prevent injury and keep you flexible. Flexibility is important to your mobility as you age.

IMPROVE YOUR MUSCLES' ABILITY TO USE INSULIN

Type 2 diabetes, also called adult-onset diabetes, is one of the most common chronic diseases around the world, affecting more than 100 million people. In the United States alone, more than 14 million people have type 2 diabetes. This disorder occurs when the body can't make enough insulin—a hormone that helps cells use or store the sugar (glucose) derived from food—or when cells and tissues can't use insulin properly. The insulin-making cells in the pancreas respond by producing more and more insulin, but they eventually can't make enough insulin to keep the blood sugar in a normal range.

People with diabetes tend to have elevated levels of blood pressure and LDL cholesterol, two major risk factors for heart disease and stroke. At the same time, the high levels of glucose in the bloodstream substantially increase the risk for developing a number of other serious medical conditions, including kidney failure, skin ulcers, limb amputation, nerve disorders, and vision disorders, including glaucoma, cataract, and blindness.

Fortunately, exercise has been shown to improve cells' sensitivity to insulin. This is true for people who have been diagnosed with type 2 diabetes as well as for those who are free from this disorder. The greater sensitivity to insulin that follows exercise can last up to 72 hours. By improving cells' ability to use insulin, exercise all by itself can also lower insulin levels in people who are overweight, even without weight loss. Exercise also replaces fat tissue with muscle tissue, which is more metabolically active and uses insulin more efficiently than fat tissue. Even moderate-intensity exercise, such as walking, can lower the risk of type 2 diabetes.

REDUCE AND REDISTRIBUTE BODY FAT

Whether you are shaped like an apple or a pear has an impact on your chances of developing heart disease. Women whose extra pounds tend to settle in the chest and waist ("apples") are more likely to have heart attacks and other heart problems and to develop diabetes than women whose extra pounds settle around their hips ("pears"). This may occur because excess fat in the chest, waist, and abdomen decreases the body's sensitivity to insulin and increases blood pressure and cholesterol levels.

For example, as the Nurses' Health Study recently demonstrated, women with a waist-to-hip ratio of 0.88 or greater were three times more likely to have developed coronary heart disease over an eight-year period than those with a waist-to-hip ratio of less than 0.72. (Calculating this ratio is simple—measure your waist at the navel—"belly button"—and your hips where they are largest, and divide the waist measurement by the hip measurement.) This trend held even for women who were not overweight.

Fortunately, you can goad your body into redistributing body fat over time, and even melt some of it away. How? With moderate ac-

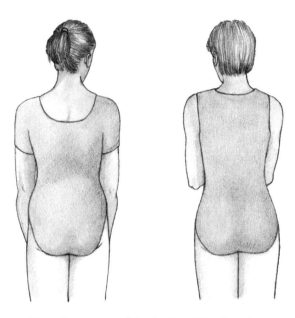

Two Patterns of Body Fat Distribution

tivity such as walking, swimming, bicycling, or whatever you choose, as long as it is done regularly and in conjunction with a healthy diet. Weight loss usually involves reductions in waist measurements and abdominal fat, often leading to a lower waist-to-hip ratio.

PREVENT CANCER

Dozens of studies have shown that people with low levels of physical activity have a higher risk of developing colon cancer, while active people have a lower risk. Similar associations have been found for breast cancer. While no one has been able to fully explain the biological mechanisms behind the apparent protective effect of exercise in these two cases, it may be due to the positive effect that physical activity has on the immune system, or to hormonal changes, or to other physiological changes that aren't yet identified. In the case of colon cancer, the mechanism could be the faster transit of food through the digestive system among active people; there's less time for carcinogens to damage the lining of the intestines. According to results from the Nurses' Health Study, moderate activity for an hour a day provides the same protection against colon cancer as vigorous activity for half an hour per day.

IMPROVE EMOTIONAL WELL-BEING

Regular physical activity produces chemical changes in the brain that improve mood, lower anxiety, and reduce symptoms of depression. When exercise is done with another person or a group, it can provide social interactions that may have a positive effect on mental health. And by promoting weight loss and muscle tone, regular activity can improve a woman's image of her own body and engender a sense of mastery that may increase self-esteem.

LESSEN THE EFFECTS OF AGING

Physical activity can dramatically improve an older person's quality of life. Stronger muscles and more flexible joints help preserve mobility and independence. Regular activity maintains basal metabolism, digestion, and circulation, while improving cognitive function, reaction time, and short-term memory. Exercise also helps to ease sleep, improve mood, and reduce anxiety and depression, which often are major problems for the elderly as they suffer losses of family and friends and their own health declines.

Don't Forget Stretching and Strength Training

The Surgeon General's report on *Physical Fitness and Health* recommends two strength-training sessions a week that include at least 8 to 10 strength-developing exercises using the major muscle groups of the legs, trunk, and shoulders, with one or two sets of 8–12 repetitions of each exercise. Strength training is important for young, middle-aged, and elderly women alike. Even 90-year-olds can make impressive strength gains with a moderate program.

Interest in strength-training seems to be on the upswing. "Attitudes toward strength training have changed from just a few years ago in many ways," says Wayne Westcott, Ph.D., a nationally recognized strength-training researcher who is based at the South Shore YMCA in Quincy, Massachusetts. "We've seen some important research for middle-aged and senior women which has emphasized the importance of not only building muscle but replacing bone. Women now know they need to maintain lean body mass to maintain their weight. They're also much more aware of osteoporosis—they know that strength training helps to prevent this devastating degenerative disease."

In one survey Westcott conducted, 75% of the older respondents who did strength training reported that they do it for health-related reasons—to help prevent heart disease, osteoporosis, diabetes, and low-back pain. "In addition," he says, "younger women see strength training as a way of improving their physical appearance, and perhaps their performance in sports activities. Women of all ages understand that strength training will help them look better and improve their health."

Here, briefly, are six good reasons to include strength training and stretching in your weekly activity regimen:

- To keep your metabolism humming
- To lose weight successfully and healthily
- To develop strong, dense bones
- To retain mobility and prevent injury
- To improve mood and ward off anxiety and depression
- To enhance your appearance

KEEP YOUR METABOLISM HUMMING

Unless you're one of the lucky ones, you've probably noticed some middle-aged spread of your very own. Barring any medical conditions, this weight gain is probably related to a changing ratio of muscle to fat. Starting in mid-life, the average woman loses five pounds of muscle each decade and adds 15 pounds of fat, for a net weight gain of ten pounds, or a pound each year. Because fatty storage tissue uses up less energy than muscle, this shift from muscle to fat slows metabolism, making it harder and harder to burn off calories. On top of that, the calories that once went into keeping muscle tissue functioning now end up going into even more fat storage. It's an unhealthy, and fattening, cycle.

Strength training can help break this cycle. Not only does a good workout stimulate muscle growth, but it also helps raise resting metabolism. To maintain itself, a pound of muscle burns up substantially more calories each day than a pound of fat. Adding new muscle (and, by extension, losing old fat) further shifts the balance in favor of calorie burning. You also use more calories during a workout and for several hours after you've finished. This combination of factors makes it easier and easier to maintain your weight as you become stronger, rather than harder to do so.

LOSE WEIGHT SUCCESSFULLY AND HEALTHILY

Say you've decided to lose those extra pounds. But, as you know, statistics on weight loss aren't encouraging. Most people—95%, in fact—have difficulty keeping weight off once they lose it. Muscle loss is a key reason. Dieting without exercising guarantees the loss of both muscle and fat. Yet when that weight is regained, as it so often is, it is invariably regained as fat tissue, not muscle tissue. This shifts the ratio of fat to muscle in your body farther toward the fat side, making you worse off than before you started dieting!

A case in point is talk show host and actress Oprah Winfrey. Using a liquid diet, she shed 69 pounds in just a few months, dropping from 211 pounds to 142 pounds. On her famous "diet show," she donned a pair of size 10 jeans and triumphantly pulled a wagon of fat behind her into the studio. The very next day, she weighed in at 145 pounds; in two weeks she was up to 155. From there her weight climbed to 237 pounds. In her book, *Make the Connection,* Oprah writes, "What I didn't know was that I had lost muscle weight. I wasn't exercising, and I didn't exercise after losing the weight. There was nothing my body could do but gain weight."

Starting a program of moderate exercise can slow this trend, and adding in some strength training can stop or even reverse it. A 12-week study performed at the University of Massachusetts Medical School clearly demonstrated that combining aerobic exercise and strength training is the best way to keep your muscles intact during a weight-loss program, helping to ensure that the fat you lose will stay off. The study compared weight loss and changes in body composition—body fat and lean muscle tissue—in 65 women, some of whom followed a moderate diet (with 30% fat or less), some of whom combined the same diet with aerobic exercise, and some of whom combined the diet with aerobic exercise and strength training.

The women who only dieted lost an average of 9 pounds, 11% of which was muscle. The women who dieted and performed aerobic exercise lost an average of 10 pounds, 99% of which was fat. The women who dieted, performed aerobic exercise, and strength trained lost an average of 13 pounds of fat. They also added 4% in new muscle. And because muscle is more metabolically active than fat, this extra muscle mass and decreased fat mass helped them burn more calories with everything that they did. So they are the *least* likely to gain back the weight they lost.

The women who did aerobic exercise (but no strength training) along with dieting lost weight and managed to preserve the muscle they had, so they have at least a fighting chance of maintaining their desired weight in the future. But the women who only dieted lost weight and muscle. As result, they are the *most likely* of any of the women in this study to regain the weight they lost at some time in the future.

DEVELOP STRONG, DENSE BONES

It is never too early or too late for a woman to start thinking about her bones, from the teenager who needs to concentrate on building as much bone as she can to the older woman interested in preventing more bone loss.

Strength training adds enough mechanical stress to help stimulate new bone growth. This is true if you are 40, 50, 60, or even 70 and have led a fairly sedentary lifestyle up until now. Strength training combined with regular physical activity, calcium supplements, vitamin D, and (for some women) hormone replacement therapy or other medication may help to slow bone loss in your spine and pelvis even after menopause.

RETAIN MOBILITY AND PREVENT INJURY

The combination of strength training, flexibility exercises, and stretching will help preserve your strength, range of motion, and balance. If you let these slip, you may be setting yourself up for a fall, literally. In a young or middle-aged woman, a fall usually isn't a big deal. But in an older women, a fall often means a fractured hip which, in turn, can require a long recovery period, sometimes with deadly complications. And even among women lucky enough not to break bones, weaker and less flexible muscles may mean that they have trouble doing simple, everyday activities such as climbing stairs, getting in and out of bed or a car, or crossing streets without assistance.

As you get older, your muscles tend to stiffen a bit, losing some of the spring that allowed them to contract, extend, and relax so easily when you were younger. Special secretions that lubricate muscle also dry up. And all this occurs on top of the progressive age-related loss of muscle we've been describing. Moving a particular muscle or muscle group, either passively with stretching or actively with weights, increases blood flow to tissues and helps keep them as functional as possible.

If you don't routinely use a muscle to its full capacity, you give up part of its range. For example, if you don't keep your neck muscles flexible, you will lose some of the range of motion in your neck and as a consequence will end up having to turn your whole body to see something beside or behind you. If your leg and back muscles lose their strength and normally lightning-fast ability to counter a sudden imbalance, falls are more likely to occur.

IMPROVE MOOD AND WARD OFF ANXIETY AND DEPRESSION

Maria Fiatarone, M.D., working at the Hebrew Rehabilitation Center for the Aged in Boston, noticed that strength training seemed to improve the mood of some of the older people with whom she was working. So she and her colleagues tested the effect of strength training on mood in a group of 32 clinically depressed people between the ages of 60 and 84. Half were assigned to discussion groups, the other half to strength-training sessions. All participants felt better after three months, largely due to the attention they received, but the improvements were greatest among those who did strength training. As a bonus, their strength increased by one third, while muscle strength in the talk-only group declined.

We don't know if the people in the strength-training group felt better because they were stronger, or if the strength training itself caused positive biochemical changes in their brains—the researchers concluded that the positive changes were due to a combination of factors.

ENHANCE YOUR APPEARANCE

Who wouldn't like to look better? As we discuss in Chapter 13, most American women—and indeed women around the world—report feeling unsatisfied with the way they look. Exercise—both aerobic activity and strength training—can help you feel more comfortable with your appearance, in part from knowing that you are doing what you can to be your best. Physical activity can help you maintain a healthy weight or lose weight over time if you need to, which for most of us would be an appearance improver. What's more, strong muscles will give your body a new shape and tone and make your clothes fit and feel better.

Adding It All Up

Let's try, then, to quantify the health benefits of regular exercise. Taking results from the many available studies into account (see Chapter 11 for more detail), we conclude that physical activity confers the following health benefits:

▪ **Premature death**	Reduces risk 30% to 50%
▪ **Heart disease**	Reduces risk 40% to 50%
▪ **Stroke**	Reduces risk 30% to 50%
▪ **Blood pressure**	Lowers blood pressure
▪ **Cholesterol**	Lowers LDL and triglycerides
	Raises HDL
▪ **Obesity**	Helps with weight reduction
	Reduces abdominal fat
	Increases metabolism and muscle mass
▪ **Diabetes (Type 2)**	Reduces risk 30% to 40%
	Improves blood sugar control
▪ **Breast cancer**	Reduces risk 20% to 30%
▪ **Colon cancer**	Reduces risk 30% to 50%
▪ **Osteoporosis**	Reduces risk 40% to 50%
▪ **Depression/anxiety**	Lowers depression and anxiety
	Relieves stress
	Improves mood

- **Emotional well-being**   Increases energy level
Improves body image
Improves outlook on life

What Happens If You Stop Exercising?

As you might have guessed, the benefits you reap from both aerobic activity and strength training dwindle soon after you stop working out. Many of the gains from aerobic exercise are lost in as little as two weeks, with the balance of the training effect fading away over 2 to 8 months. The extra strength you've gotten from strength training may last for 4 to 6 weeks but will slip away after that.

Points to Remember

- In this book, fitness refers to functional fitness rather than cardio-respiratory fitness. The 30 minutes of aerobic exercise that we suggest you do each day will strengthen your heart and lungs; help you maintain bone mass, muscle strength, and flexibility; improve the way your body responds to insulin and handles blood sugar; reduce and help redistribute body fat; improve digestive efficiency; enhance your emotional well-being; and lessen the effects of aging. It won't, however, prepare you to run a marathon or engage in other vigorous sports.
- Two sessions of strength training per week will keep your metabolism in tune and maintain your weight or help you lose weight successfully. It will also preserve or add muscle and bone mass, enhance your mobility, protect you from injury, improve your emotional well-being, and make you look better and feel better about your appearance.
- If you stop exercising, these benefits will begin to fade within 2 weeks and most will vanish over a 2–8-month period.

"It is good to have an end to journey towards; but it is the
journey that matters in the end."

Ursula Le Guin (1929–), science fiction writer

3

Four Steps to a New Exercise Habit: An Overview

For better or for worse, polls take the pulse of the nation. They offer us a peek at what we like and don't like, what we do and don't do, what we have and what we want. Several recent polls suggest that the American pulse is beating on the lethargic side when it comes to physical activity. Most American adults don't exercise regularly. The good news is that polls can help explain why, and what can be done about it.

One such national opinion survey, "American Attitudes Toward Physical Activity and Fitness," was commissioned by the President's Council on Physical Fitness and Sports and the Sporting Goods Manufacturers' Association. This 1993 telephone survey of 1,018 "less active adults" age 18 and older examined how interested these people were in increasing their physical activity and what barriers they thought existed to doing so. For the purposes of this poll, less active people were defined as those who engaged in vigorous exercise less than twice a week.

The poll showed a surprising amount of interest in exercise, as well as some clear choices in favor of physical activity that might not be considered exercise—activities such as gardening and dancing. A majority of respondents (59%) said they wanted to become more active, and 49% said they thought it would be easy to increase their activity level. In addition, 41% said they were aware of a link

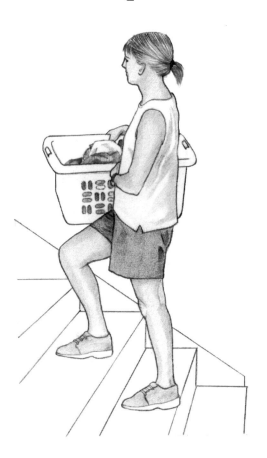

between regular physical activity and improved health and appearance.

If people have the knowledge concerning the benefits of exercise, and the desire to exercise, then why don't they *just do it?* Lack of time, said 64% of the respondents, with nearly half reporting they had less than 10 hours of leisure time per week. Yet 84% reported watching more than three hours of television a week. (In other words, they have the time to exercise, but they prefer to do other things instead.)

Another survey—a 1995 poll of 1,000 people age 18 and older commissioned by former U.S. Surgeon General C. Everett Koop's "Shape Up, America!" campaign—showed that Americans are discouraged about becoming more active because they view exercise as being too hard and too time-consuming. This poll suggests that part of the problem stems from some rather outdated notions about exercise and health.

One of our main goals of this book is to demonstrate that exercise need not be either difficult or time-consuming to be beneficial—and rewarding.

What's Stopping You?

Women and girls face unique obstacles when it comes to exercise. Karrie Donovan, a personal trainer and fitness consultant, says that many women she has worked with never had any experience with athletics when they were young, and so they often don't feel confident about starting an activity later in life. Mary, a 59-year-old florist, is a prime example. When she began exercising soon after her 40th birthday, the experience was a new one, since she grew up with very little encouragement toward physical activity. "Tetherball was the only thing I played in grade school and junior high," she says. "In high school I didn't do anything. Sports were for boys; it was something I never questioned. I played baseball in gym class with girls, but there was no support. Girls were kind of ignored. The message was that physical activity wasn't for us. While I am happy that I appreciate exercise now, at the same time I'm just sick about the fact that it took me so long to appreciate it because I enjoy exercise and it has helped me so much."

The situation may be completely different for our daughters and granddaughters. The landmark 1972 law commonly referred to as Title IX opened the door to wider participation in school sports for women. In many communities, there are as many soccer and basketball teams for girls as there are for boys. And the thrilling victory of the United States Women's Soccer Team in capturing the 1999 Women's World Cup and the success of the WNBA professional women's basketball league have fired many athletic dreams and ambitions among girls and young women in this country. Together, these changes may mean that American women of the twenty-first century will be more active than their twentieth-century counterparts.

On top of the lack of emphasis on sports and physical activity for girls and women, women have traditionally been taught to put family and job responsibilities ahead of their own needs. As a result, the notion of taking personal time for exercise may elicit feelings of guilt, even though inactivity is a legitimate health issue. "The women I work with have so many other priorities—taking care of people in their lives, running a home, keeping a job outside the home—it's often hard for them to take time for themselves," says Donovan.

As a result, many of us find ourselves caught in a cycle of inactivity and weight gain throughout our lives, mostly because long-term weight management is especially difficult for inactive people. When inactive women begin losing muscle mass after age 30, their metabolism slows as the fat-to-muscle ratio shifts further and further in the direction of fat. So even when women are eating the same way they did when they were 20, this change in metabolism causes them to gain weight in middle age. The hormonal changes that accompany menopause often kick this process into overdrive if women remain inactive.

In this chapter, and in Chapters 4–7 we will demonstrate how this unfortunate cycle of inactivity and weight gain can be reversed with an intelligent, well-constructed plan that consists of moderate exercise, some simple strength-training exercises, and moderate eating.

We owe a debt of gratitude to James Annesi, Ph.D., an exercise and sports psychology consultant, researcher, instructor, and author of *Enhancing Exercise Motivation*. Dr. Annesi has studied hundreds of people just beginning exercise programs at fitness centers around the country, and he speaks with authority on what makes people stick with exercise and why they drop out. Much of the information in this chapter was derived from conversations with Dr. Annesi and from his book, as well as from our own experience with patients and colleagues.

Eliminating Mental Barriers

In order to change a habit in the first place, it is necessary to *believe that you can do it*. If you're not yet completely convinced that you can become more physically active, the mental exercise outlined in

BOX 8

What's Holding You Back?

- **Point:** I don't like to sweat.
  Counterpoint: If I just walk for 30 minutes, I probably won't sweat much. Besides, sweating is natural, and I'll treat myself to a relaxing shower or bath when I'm finished.
- **Point:** I'd like to be more active, but I don't want anyone to see me exercise.
  Counterpoint: I can find an activity I can do in the privacy of my own home—even in my own room, if necessary.
- **Point:** My family doesn't exercise, and I'll be taking time away from them if I do.
  Counterpoint: I can involve my family in my activity; it would be good for them. If they aren't interested, it will be nice to have some time for myself.
- **Point:** Physical activity is for athletes, and I'm just not an athlete.
  Counterpoint: Walking for 30 minutes is something that just about everyone can do naturally.
- **Point:** If I start to exercise, I'll develop bulky muscles, and I don't want that.
  Counterpoint: Thirty minutes of walking, or light stretching and strengthening exercises, will not give me big muscles. It *will* help me keep the muscles I have, which will help me control my weight.

- **Point:** _____

  Counterpoint: _____

- **Point:** _____

  Counterpoint: _____

- **Point:** _____

  Counterpoint: _____

If you can think of anything else that may be holding you back, fill it in above, along with your idea of what you can do about it.

Box 8 may help you identify blocks in your thinking that may impede your success. The point here is to identify the negative thoughts or doubts you may have regarding exercise and then to think of positive ways around these obstacles.

Managing the Time Crunch

For many of us, lack of time is the biggest barrier to starting an exercise program or getting more exercise. Some days it feels as though just grabbing a lunch or finding time to go to the bathroom is a major challenge; setting aside a solid half hour to walk, run, bike, lift weights, or whatever is out of the question.

There's a way out of this bind. Some exciting new research suggests that you can get just as many benefits from several short bouts of activity sprinkled throughout the day as you can from one long session. This approach, called *intermittent exercise,* may work even better for some women because it is more convenient and so more doable. Take, for example, a 1999 study in the *Journal of the American Medical Association* by Rena R. Wing, Ph.D., and other investigators. Dr. Wing is internationally recognized for her research on behavioral approaches to obesity and weight loss. She and her colleagues assigned 148 volunteers, all of whom were sedentary, overweight women, to one of three exercise schedules done five days a week—one 40-minute session a day, four 10-minute sessions a day without exercise equipment, or four 10-minute sessions with exercise equipment (a motorized treadmill at home). At six months, women in all three groups had lost roughly the same amount of weight, about 17 pounds. At 18 months, though, those who were doing short bouts of exercise and had access to treadmills at home had managed to keep all that weight off, while women in the other two groups were gradually regaining weight. What's more, 88% of the women with access to a treadmill were still exercising at 18 months, compared with about 70% in the other two groups.

This doesn't mean you need to rush out and buy an expensive treadmill or other type of indoor exercise machine. An exercise video you can pop in the VCR and work out with for 10 or 15 minutes would probably do just as well. Instead, the take-home message from this study is that short bouts of exercise add up. If you can't carve half an hour out of your days, then 10- or 15-minute chunks will do just fine.

Changing Old Habits

As the Surgeon General's report on *Physical Activity and Health* makes clear, poor lifestyle habits are responsible for an estimated 300,000 deaths per year in America. For that reason, physicians, public health officials, behavioral scientists, and others have thought long and hard about the nature of lifestyle change. Because smoking leads the pack in terms of the number of people it kills and injures, the process by which people stop—or try to stop—smoking has received close scrutiny.

When the first Surgeon General's report conclusively linked smoking to lung cancer and heart disease in 1964, half of adult men and more than one third of adult women smoked. Today, only about one quarter of adult men and women smoke. That reduction is due, in part, to some major changes of attitude in our society. Thanks to 40 years of public education campaigns, people are now more aware of the hazards of smoking, and it has lost some of its glamour and mystique. Opportunities to smoke are rarer than they used to be: smoking has been banned on airlines and in many restaurants and other public places. And there are fewer stimuli to take up the habit of smoking: ads for cigarettes can no longer appear in newspapers or on outdoor billboards. Influenced by these changes, millions of smokers have made the difficult personal decision to quit. Many of them actually follow through on this decision, though only a minority achieve their goal.

Changing a habit of inactivity is much like stopping smoking. So a number of researchers have tried to adapt much of what we've learned over the years about smoking to exercise behavior. One useful approach is the five stages of change for smoking cessation devised by James Prochaska, professor of clinical and health psychology at the University of Rhode Island, and adapted to exercise by Bess Marcus, associate professor of psychiatry and human behavior at Brown University. See if you can recognize your own "exercise stage" in the list below:

- **Precontemplation:** During this stage, the person is not yet active or is yet not thinking about making a change. She has probably not exercised on her own or worked out in a fitness facility.
- **Contemplation:** The person is not active but wants to be. She has some barriers to exercise and is not yet ready to begin an exercise program. However, she might be buying fitness books and tapes or reading reports in newspapers or magazines about exercise to gather the information needed to get started.
- **Preparation:** The person is starting to exercise, but her efforts are still sporadic. She understands the importance of regular exercise but has not yet established a regular habit.
- **Action:** The person exercises regularly but has not yet done so for six months—the time it takes to form a durable exercise habit.
- **Maintenance:** The person has been exercising regularly for six months or more.

According to Drs. Prochaska and Marcus, if you can identify a person's stage of change, you can give her the information, support, and tools needed to move to the next stage. Clearly, just the fact that you're making the effort to read this book indicates that you're well past the precontemplation phase. You're aware that you need to exercise, and you've decided to take some steps to get going.

Perhaps the most critical step is that of exchanging the habit of not exercising for the habit of exercising. In other words, replacing something you already do—like watching television—with some kind of physical activity. Giving up an old habit that is comfortable and familiar for a new one that may be somewhat uncomfortable at the beginning will probably require a little bit of mental and behavioral reprogramming.

If you've ever written someone's old address on an envelope months after they've moved, or written a check dated last year, you know how durable the simplest habit can be. Sooner or later, though, as you remind yourself of the change, the old habit fades and is eventually replaced by a new one, albeit with a few missteps along the way. A similar process occurs when you begin establishing an activity habit. Initially, you gravitate to the old habit and have to remind yourself to exercise. With practice, though, your new exercise habit becomes imbedded in your memory and your muscles, gradually becoming more familiar and easier to execute.

Once you've established an exercise habit, the small choices you have to make every day to be active will become second nature. Obstacles will still arise periodically to challenge that habit—your schedule may change because you or your partner takes a new job, your child changes schools, you move to a new neighborhood, or you begin caring for an aging parent. You may find that you've slid backward from the action stage to the preparation stage. Not to worry. If you lapse for a time, it's important to see the lapse as momentary rather than as a failure or a character flaw. Because lapses in an exercise routine are a normal part of life, in Chapter 7 we've included some helpful tools that you can use to get back on track.

Making the Transition from Inactive to Active

Old lifestyle habits tend to fit us like comfortable shoes—whether they're good for us or not. We stick with them because they've become familiar and they conform to our lives. Because most of us don't like change very much, forming a new habit is a challenging process. During a transition from old to new, we have to give up the comfort and familiarity of the old behavior in favor of a new practice that can feel terribly foreign. We experience this discomfort until the new practice becomes the lifestyle-equivalent of a comfortable old shoe.

People who succeed in making the change from inactivity to regular activity have the ability to withstand this kind of minor discomfort until the new habit forms, something that can take between 3 and 6 months. Early in the process, a sort of mental balance sheet forms in the mind. At first it is rather heavily weighted on the negative side—toward what we're giving up. Ever so gradually, though, it shifts toward the positives—the rewards we get from the new activity.

For example, let's say you want to spend less money and save more. In return for not buying whatever you want whenever you want it, you will get a fatter savings account and more financial security. Exercising fiscal restraint initially yields only deprivation—at first, whenever you see an attractive item in a store, you may feel a twinge of deprivation each time you discipline yourself not to take out your credit card or cash. Little by little, though, as your savings account builds, the negative feeling of being deprived becomes outweighed by the positive feeling of dollars and interest accumulating in your savings account. If you can live with the discomfort of fiscal restraint long enough to make it a habit, way down the road you'll be rewarded by having money for a downpayment on a house, or college tuition for the kids, or a comfortable retirement. The key is sticking with your plan until your balance sheet has shifted toward the payoff. This type of self-discipline will enable you to reach just about any goal.

So it goes with exercise. Say you decide to start walking in the morning. That means going to bed earlier the night before (if possible) and maybe waking up at sunrise. You may feel a little out of place exercising outdoors in plain view of your neighbors. You may feel a little winded and your legs may get sore, especially if your route is hilly. You'll probably wonder why you are doing this when you could be sleeping in a warm bed. The balance sheet is clearly in the red.

But after a week or two or four, you'll begin to see—and feel—the payoff. You may find that you actually *enjoy* getting up earlier. You may meet a few of your early-bird neighbors. The soreness in your legs will go away, and you'll discover you aren't getting winded any longer. The sense of mastery and control you get from your daily walk may brighten up each day. Within a month (or two), you may begin to see improvements in your fitness, some toning in your legs, and even a small weight loss. These changes add to your sense of pride (see Box 9).

The key to success is to stick to your plan until your balance sheet shifts away from the feeling that you're missing something—like a half hour of sleep—toward the feeling that you've gained something. Maybe it's the pleasure of strolling through a quiet, just-waking neighborhood. Or a sunset over the pond you like to walk around. Or maybe it's the pleasure of people-watching as you walk down a busy street at lunchtime. Finally, knowing that you are doing a wonderful thing to safeguard your own health can have a tremendously positive effect on your self-esteem.

BOX 9

A Sample Exercise Balance Sheet

Activity	Time frame	Negatives	Positives
A.M. walk	Weeks 1–2	Less sleep; feel out of place; mild leg soreness; feel winded	Sense of pride; enjoyment of morning
A.M. walk	Weeks 3–4	Less sleep; still feel out of place; no physiological changes yet apparent	Sense of pride; enjoyment of morning; soreness gone; less winded
A.M. walk	Weeks 5–8	Less sleep	Sense of pride; enjoyment of morning; more comfortable doing activity; first signs of toning in legs; small weight loss; improved functional fitness

The Four Steps: Plan, Proceed, Record, Reward

Because changing your behavior involves some discomfort, at least initially, you'll need to give yourself some reasonable, attainable goals to start with. Expecting to adopt an exercise habit overnight isn't practical. What's more, it isn't being fair to yourself. Jumping full-steam-ahead into a new activity program would probably make exercise seem like a frustrating burden. It wouldn't give you enough time to rearrange your schedule appropriately and would overload you both mentally and physically.

It's much better to make this transition in a steady, methodical manner, increasing your exercise in "spoonfuls" so you can get used to this new, acquired taste. If you plan to exercise first thing in the morning, your goal for the first week might be getting to bed earlier on just two or three nights so you can get up earlier the following mornings and exercise. Once you've accomplished that goal, try it again the next week, and the next, adding a third, fourth, and then fifth day until pretty soon you've built yourself an excellent exercise routine.

We describe our four-step process in detail in Chapter 4 (planning your active lifestyle), Chapter 5 (proceeding with your exercise program), Chapter 6 (recording your progress), and Chapter 7 (rewarding your efforts), and briefly outline these points below. Reading through these steps will take very little of your time, and it will help you create a vision of your new exercise habit in your mind. It will also help you focus on your growing positive feelings about exercise, feelings that will help get you through the early months of your program.

STEP 1: PLAN YOUR ACTIVITY

As a general rule, the more active you are, the more healthy you will become. In Chapter 4 we discuss the relationship of exercise to an active lifestyle. You may have particular goals in addition to overall health that you want to accomplish through your exercise session, such as weight loss or getting your body ready to play a particular sport; we'll discuss how much exercise you need in order to accomplish your goals. We'll help you decide on a type of exercise that suits your personality and encourage you to monitor your exercise intensity so you can always determine if you're exercising at a safe level of exertion. Finally, we'll try to dispel some myths about strength training, an important activity that many women tend to overlook. And we'll give you some suggestions for finding often overlooked pockets of time in your busy schedule that you can use for exercise.

STEP 2: PROCEED TO EXERCISE

You'll never know if you're making progress if you don't know where you started. Exercise physiologists call this starting point the baseline. Chapter 5 begins with some simple tests you can take to determine your baseline fitness level. It also contains a "Personal Goal Profile" that will help you further determine your baseline goals and your movement toward them. The "Exercise-Induced Feeling Inventory" will measure how happy, energetic, tired out, and so on you're feeling, so that later you can compare this baseline with your feelings after you've exercised.

We also give you tips for starting a walking program, plus some practical pointers for getting started on that very first day. This chapter also contains information about starting a strength-training program, and refers you to Chapter 8, where we give the details of three indoor exercise programs: a "15-Minute Strength Essentials" program that emphasizes functional fitness; a "20-minute Total Body Basics" program that will help you build some strength; and a "20-minute Quick Intervals" program that combines cardiovascular and strength-training in one. In Chapter 8 we also present some simple stretching exercises that we encourage you to do twice a day.

STEP 3: RECORD (MONITOR) YOUR PROGRESS

Blame it on grammar school report cards or annual reviews, but many of us find that knowing where we stand and how we're doing helps us keep on track. The same is true for starting to exercise. Whatever activity you've chosen, we suggest that you keep a log, like the ones in Chapter 6, of how often you exercise and for how long. We also suggest that you record your mood using the "Exercise-Induced Feeling Inventory" before and after your activity to help you become aware of the mood-elevating benefits of physical activity. Or, if you prefer, record your activity—and your feelings before and after exercise—in the daily schedule planner that you use to keep track of all your important appointments. You might also try putting a large monthly calendar on your refrigerator or closet door and recording on it your results and changing moods. That way, you can look at an entire month's effort in a glance and see what you've accomplished and how you're progressing.

STEP 4: REWARD YOUR EFFORT

After you've finished your workout, do something that you enjoy—take a bubble bath or hot shower, fix yourself a cup of coffee or a cappuccino and read a chapter of a good novel, treat yourself to a professional massage at the end of the week or some other relaxation treat of your choosing. Fantasize about how you'll reward yourself once you've completed three months, six months, a full year of exercise.

At the very least, take a few moments after your workout to put your feet up and give yourself credit for what you've just done. Many people make the mistake of mindlessly pushing themselves through a workout, then immediately moving on to the next task. Instead, we hope you will work out *mindfully,* paying particular attention to how your mood improves as you exercise, then give yourself time to feel good about what you've accomplished. These suggestions are just other ways to get you to focus *on the good feelings that exercise brings about.* Experiencing and acknowledging these feelings are important steps in shifting your internal balance sheet in favor of the positives. You will also be able to recall the good feelings on a difficult day and use them to get yourself through it. Do that successfully over a period of months and you will have established a durable exercise habit.

Why Four Steps?

You may be wondering if all of this is necessary. That depends on the individual. If you are already motivated to start exercising and committed to following through, then you can try skimming these chapters. But please don't hurry over the sections in Chapter 5 that contain information on walking and strength training. We think you will also find the logs in Chapter 5 that track how much and how often you exercise to be very helpful.

Most women (and men, too!) need a careful plan such as the one we've laid out to set themselves up for success. Fitness trainer Karrie Donovan, for example, helped her own 50-year-old mother plan her exercise routine: "I knew that my mom would need some structure and some built-in reward to exercise. As a preschool teacher, she rarely gets to watch Regis Philbin in the morning. So I suggested that she program her VCR to tape their show every day while she is at school. Then, when she comes home, she can pop the tape into the VCR and watch it while she uses her cross-country ski machine. When she started, I suggested that she do it for 20 minutes. Now, she's up to 30."

A number of things about this routine helped make it a success. First, Donovan's mom *planned* her exercise for the end of her day when she knew she'd have time and needed to unwind and perk up. She keeps her ski machine where she knows she will really use it—near the television. And she rewards herself by exercising while she watches her favorite program, something she looks forward to during the day.

"I know my mom's main motivation was to lose the few pounds that she gained around her waist during menopause, and she's done that," Donovan explains. "I know she also wants to keep her bones strong. In addition, her workout helps her regain some energy she loses during the day. She often comes home exhausted after spending the day with a room full of four-year-olds."

Focus on Positive Feelings

At this point, we'd like to clarify an issue that is very important to the success of any new exercise program. When most of us exercise, we expect results—some definite, observable change that occurs because of our efforts. When it comes to exercise, there are two types of results—physiological and psychological.

Physiological results include weight loss, toned muscles, a smaller waist, hips, or thighs, and improvements in functional fitness such as being less winded when you climb stairs, a greater tolerance for physical activity, or a slower heartbeat. Psychological changes include reduced stress, improved mood, increased energy, a greater sense of control over your life, and deeper, more restful sleep.

But physiological and psychological results don't necessarily happen at the same time, which can be confusing and even frustrating. Psychological changes are likely to occur almost immediately, while physiological changes often take months to occur and may initially fool you by heading in the wrong direction. If you are walking and strength training for example, you may see your weight tick *upward* as you add a bit of muscle. But if you keep at it, you'll start seeing some pounds melt away.

"It can be frustrating," says sport psychologist James Annesi, "when a person starts to feel very good from a psychological standpoint about their exercise program but doesn't yet see any physiological changes. He or she may begin to feel energetic and trim, and thus expect to see weight loss reflected on the scale. A problem may result if those high expectations aren't realized."

To get around this common barrier, we urge you to focus on your *perception* of the benefits of your exercise program. Listen to how you are feeling, and don't let your feelings be squelched by what the scale is saying. One way to do this is to use the "Personal Goal Profile" and the "Exercise-Induced Feeling Inventory" often. If you acknowledge the good feelings—reductions in stress and improvements in mood—as progress, you'll continue with exercise and you'll begin to lock in an exercise habit that will ultimately pay off with weight loss and many other benefits.

Joan, a 38-year-old lawyer, used exercise to help her cope with the stress of her first job in a big law firm. "When I started practicing law, there was a tremendous amount of pressure to perform. I was working long hours and worrying about everything. Soon after starting with this firm, I joined a gym. It was a struggle to fit in the time for a workout, but it was well worth the effort. Working on the strength machines, or lifting light free weights, or stair climbing helped me get rid of some of my frustration and anxiety. I rarely thought about work while exercising, which was a great relief. It really helped me handle the stress that seemed to keep building up in my life."

Find a Source of Support

Creating an exercise habit on your own is a challenge. While some of you will be content to do so with the tools contained in this book, others of you will want additional outside support.

If you need support, try getting your partner or a friend involved in your activity plan. Doing so will not only help you stick with your program but it will also be beneficial to his or her health. A 1996 study published in the *Journal of Sports Medicine and Physical Fitness,* for example, reported that married people who joined a fitness program as a couple had significantly higher attendance and adherence rates than married people who joined by themselves. Both the married pairs and married singles had the same levels of self-motivation, so the higher attendance and adherence in married pairs may have been due to the social support and camaraderie provided by an exercising partner.

If your "significant other" isn't interested, or you could never coordinate your exercise schedules, support from other exercisers and staff members is usually available at health clubs and YMCAs. Such clubs also offer exercise instruction, and many have day care facilities and exercise centers for children that are included in the membership or are available for a small additional fee. If a fitness membership doesn't fit your style or your budget, ask a neighbor or friend—better yet, several neighbors or friends—to exercise with you. You'll be surprised how quickly your exercise time can elapse when it is accompanied by conversation with an exercise partner. Or follow some of the ideas outlined in Box 10.

BOX 10

Ten Ways to Support Your Activity Effort

- Find a walking/exercise buddy.
- Be the one in your household who walks the dog (or do it as a family).
- Find new activities to do—biking, hiking, swimming, and so on— to add variety.
- Combine walking time with family time when possible.
- Walk for a good cause.
- Establish a walking club in your neighborhood.
- Find a walking trail, or other venue, for weekends.
- Trade child care with a neighbor so you can both have time to walk.
- Join a community walking program at the park and recreation department, YMCA/YWCA, or health club.
- Create a vacation around walking or hiking in a new place you'd like to explore.

It is our hope that this book will help you give yourself the gift of physical fitness every day from now on. We use the word *gift* here in several ways. In one sense, taking the time for physical activity each day is a little break from your hectic routine, and this brief breather is a small gift you give yourself; the health benefits you'll get are a much larger gift for you and the people you love. A gift is also defined as a notable capacity, talent, or endowment, something that physical activity, exercise, and participation in sports can become over time.

So many of life's events are beyond our control—a child's illness in the middle of the night, sudden changes at work, a fender-bender during rush hour, the unexpected death of a family member or close friend. We can, however, exert some control over our lifestyles and habits. Simple changes made on a daily basis, such as choosing to exercise and eat healthier food, can help us wrest control out of what may seem to be chaos and give our lives a sense of order that may have eluded us before.

Points to Remember

- You are not destined to be inactive. Even if you've been sedentary for most of your life, you don't have to continue living this way if you don't want to.
- You don't need a lot of time to become more active. If you are looking to improve your health, several short (10- to 15-minute) bursts of exercise are the equivalent of the 30 minutes daily suggested by the Surgeon General.
- You don't have to be an athlete to start a regular activity program. If you choose a simple, natural activity like walking, you'll catch on within a few weeks. Even slightly more complex activities such as a light aerobics class will become second nature after a few workouts.
- You don't need to do vigorous or strenuous exercise to reap health benefits—even brisk walking can dramatically improve your health.
- You don't have to enjoy an activity right off the bat to begin developing an exercise habit. That will come later, as you begin to feel

successful with your new program. You can, indeed *learn* to enjoy physical activity.

- Don't wait around for motivation to strike. Action breeds motivation, so get moving. The simplest things can motivate you, just as the simplest things can thwart you from your goal. Sometimes the smallest act—something as mundane as putting on your sneakers or exercise clothes—may be all you need to get started.

"It's not just enough to swing at the ball. You've got to loosen your girdle and let 'er fly."

"Babe" Didrikson Zaharias (1914–1956), Olympic gold medalist and golf champion

4

Step 1: Plan Your Active Lifestyle

Creating an active lifestyle isn't complicated, and living one doesn't need to take much extra time. Simply adding some oomph to everyday tasks is an excellent start—whether you're vacuuming, commuting, chauffeuring kids, meeting with clients, or just taking a TV break.

Start by putting the "fidget factor" to work for you. This term, coined by researchers at the Mayo Clinic, comes from the astonishing and encouraging results of a study they did with the cooperation of 16 volunteers, all of whom had sedentary jobs and none of whom engaged in regular exercise. For eight days, the volunteers ate an extra 1,000 calories a day while they lived in a special metabolic unit at the Mayo Clinic that was furnished much like a regular home. Their activity levels were continually monitored, as was their blood chemistry. At the end of the study, some of the volunteers had gained as many as 16 pounds, others as few as 2. The big difference was the fidget factor—the people who gained less weight registered more activity than those who gained a lot of weight. We're not talking about exercise here, since none of the volunteers exercised during the study. We're talking about small movements such as standing up often, stretching, bouncing a leg. The researchers concluded that simply moving around requires calorie-burning muscle movement, thereby utilizing calories that might otherwise be stored as fat.

Research shows that you need to burn between 1,500 and 2,000

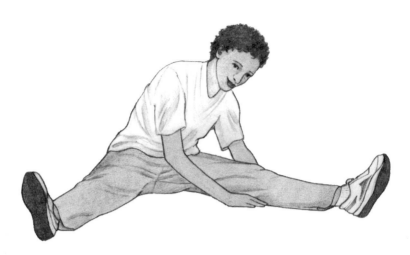

calories per week in physical activity to attain optimum health. You can easily reach that benchmark by combining a several-times-weekly exercise session of 30 minutes with other normal things you might do during the course of your day, and with recreational activities on the weekend. The idea is to look for *any and every opportunity* in your day to expend energy.

In this chapter, we will:

- Offer suggestions for adding activity to your day.
- Help you clarify your goals. Recognizing that many of you may have a specific fitness goal over and above better health, we will discuss the amount and the intensity of exercise you need to accomplish your goal.
- Help you gauge the intensity of your exercise by encouraging you to monitor your heart rate and record your MET score, a simple measure of the energy you use in doing various activities.
- Help you choose which core activity is right for your daily exercise session.
- Discuss the vital importance of strength training and stretching in helping preserve muscle and bone mass, improving your range of motion and balance, and protecting you from injury—no matter what your age.

- Consider a very practical matter—how you can fit one or more regular exercise sessions into your busy day.

Adding "Activity Bits" to Your Life

Once you begin to recognize opportunities for adding extra activity to your daily routine, you will begin to see them everywhere. The idea is to look at things you already do each day and inject them with a bit more physical energy. Not only will this help you burn extra calories but it may also spread the positive feeling that comes with exercise throughout your day. Here are some suggestions:

- **At home:** Stretch while you watch television, talk on the phone, or wait for the clothes to dry. Walk or bicycle, don't drive, to the post office to mail a letter or to the convenience store to buy bread and milk. Vacuum the rugs with vigor. Cut the grass, trim the hedges, weed the flower beds, and hoe the garden with hearty enthusiasm and hand tools rather than power tools. Shovel the driveway in the winter instead of using a snow blower. If you have a baby, break out the stroller and go for a long, brisk walk. (For mothers who want or need more activity, joggers are available for running with an infant or toddler.) Schedule walking dates with your husband and your best friend. When you walk the dog, go a bit farther and a bit faster than you ordinarily do.
- **In the car:** While waiting for a red light to change, roll your shoulders, flex your neck, and stretch your calves and your ankles. If you are on a long trip, get out of the car once an hour to walk around a rest stop or parking lot, touch your toes (gently, with knees bent), or stretch your calves while leaning against the car. Taking a fitness break will not only prevent neck and back pain later, it will also keep you more alert.
- **On the job:** Park the car at the far end of the parking lot. Skip a bus or subway stop and walk the extra distance to the office. Take the stairs instead of the elevator. Stretch your calves at the copier. Flex your back and legs and stretch your arms and back while sitting at your desk. Stretch your neck and upper back while sitting at the

computer. Instead of having your lunch delivered, walk out to get it. Better yet, try walking at lunch time, either outside around your office or indoors at a nearby shopping mall.

- **On a business trip:** Walk around the airport during layovers between flights. Choose a hotel with a fitness center. Carry a jump rope and light weights in your suitcase. Before a business meeting, relax by using a towel to stretch your arms, legs, and back. Look for an early morning exercise program on the hotel TV.
- **On vacation:** Walk, jog, bike, hike, climb, dance, golf, roller skate, ice skate, in-line skate, swim, sail, raft, kayak, canoe, windsurf, water ski, downhill ski, cross-country ski, snow shoe, or toboggan.

How does all this work in practice? Here is how Ellen, a 46-year-old working mom who decided to invest in physical activity after her mother had a heart attack, has managed to boost her energy output throughout the day. "It's a lot of little things, really. At home, I try to keep moving, especially in the evening after dinner. That used to be my TV time. I go upstairs to help my children with their homework rather than have them come down. I've been doing more of the yard work at home, something I always left to my husband or son. At work, I walk downstairs to the coffee shop instead of taking the elevator or getting a cup in the kitchen on my floor. Being aware of how little activity I used to get has made me see ways to get more, especially on the days when I know I won't get out for a long walk."

What Is Your Core Goal?

Think for a moment. Other than improved health, is there something else that's motivating you to become more physically active? You may simply want to improve your mood and energy level. You may be trying to fit into that mother-of-the-bride dress or slim that post-pregnancy belly. Or maybe you are discovering your "inner athlete" and want to begin training for more vigorous activities such as cycling, cross-country skiing, hiking, or jogging.

The benefits of exercise come from a combination of intensity, duration, and frequency; you adjust each of these factors to reach your particular goal. In the following sections we offer some guidelines for meeting three basic goals: (1) functional fitness, better long-term health, and improved mood; (2) weight loss; and (3) cardiorespiratory fitness, in preparation for more strenuous sports or activities.

LEVEL 1: FUNCTIONAL FITNESS, BETTER LONG-TERM HEALTH, AND IMPROVED MOOD

If you are sedentary now, or are active only sporadically, you can reach a level of functional fitness and reap important health benefits merely from walking briskly—or doing some other moderate activity—for a minimum of 30 minutes per day on most, preferably all, days of the week. We define walking briskly as walking a mile in 15–20 minutes; in other words, a walking rate of 3–4 miles an hour. Doing that can reduce your risk of developing heart disease by as much as 40%. It can also reduce your risk of developing type 2 diabetes, stroke, or osteoporosis. For older women, moderate activity can help guard against falls, a common cause of potentially debilitating broken bones.

Exercising for 30 minutes on most days of the week should also help reduce anxiety and improve your mood. For most people, this is long enough and often enough for your body to release chemicals called *endorphins*. These morphine-like compounds act on your brain to brighten your mood and relieve pain. If you have ever been upset, gone out to walk it off, and felt more calm and relaxed when you finished, then you already know the power of endorphins. In fact, many people find exercise so enjoyable that they get "addicted" to this relaxed feeling and miss it when they skip an exercise session.

Changes in self-esteem may begin to occur as you establish a durable exercise habit and start feeling a sense of accomplishment and increased control over your life. Feeling better about the way you look will also help raise your self-esteem. (For more on exercise, mood, and body image, see Chapter 13.)

LEVEL 2: WEIGHT LOSS

Weight gain is the result of an unbalanced energy equation—you take in more calories than you use up. Losing weight merely means reversing that equation and using more calories than you take in. As we will discuss in Chapter 10, if you combine moderate changes in your diet with 30 minutes of daily brisk walking and two 15-minute sessions of strength training per week, you will lose weight. Granted, this weight loss won't be fast, but it will be steady and durable.

If you want to lose a substantial amount of weight and you are motivated to lose it more quickly than that, research has shown that you will need to increase the duration of your exercise sessions to at least 40 to 60 minutes a day and will need to do these longer sessions four to six times per week. You may also have to increase the intensity of your activity, say from a moderately brisk walking pace (4 miles an hour) to a vigorous one (4.5 or 5 miles an hour).

Most women can safely lose up to a pound a week. There are several ways to accomplish this. To lose one pound in a week, you could either burn off the equivalent of 3,500 calories through exercise or cut out the equivalent of 3,500 calories (500 calories a day) from your diet, neither of which would be easy (see Box 11). But by combining the two—exercising a little more and eating a little less—you can achieve the same goal with much less discomfort. Any combination of calorie restriction and exercise designed so you burn more calories than you take in is the most practical and effective way to lose weight.

Exercise physiologists have devised an ingenious way to characterize energy use. Called the metabolic equivalent, or MET for short, it represents the amount of calories burned by a particular activity compared to sitting still or resting (see Box 12). Sitting still is defined as one MET, and progressively more vigorous activities have progressively higher METs. For example, brisk walking at the rate of 3.5 miles per hour is equivalent to 4 METs, meaning it uses four times as many calories as sitting still.

Burning calories is a function of three things—the MET score of an activity, how long you do the activity, and your weight. For example, a 125-pound person burns about 230 calories walking briskly for one hour (4 METs), while a 155-pound person burns close to 280 calories doing the same thing. A 125-pound person burns about 200 calories jogging at 5 miles per hour for one half hour (7 METs), while a 155-pound person burns about 250.

If you do the math, you'll see that a 155-pound woman would have

BOX 11

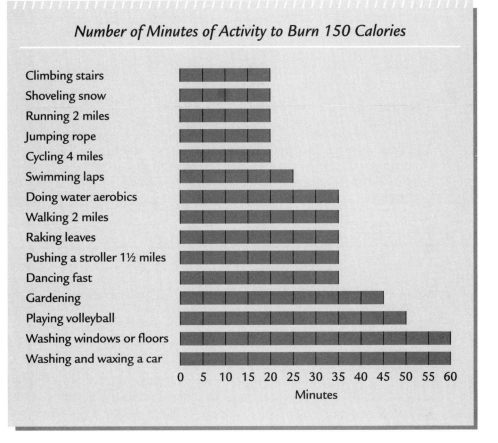

Number of Minutes of Activity to Burn 150 Calories

Activity	Minutes
Climbing stairs	
Shoveling snow	
Running 2 miles	
Jumping rope	
Cycling 4 miles	
Swimming laps	
Doing water aerobics	
Walking 2 miles	
Raking leaves	
Pushing a stroller 1½ miles	
Dancing fast	
Gardening	
Playing volleyball	
Washing windows or floors	
Washing and waxing a car	

0   5   10   15   20   25   30   35   40   45   50   55   60

Minutes

to jog for seven hours in a week, covering about 35 miles, to burn off one pound without changing her diet! Most of us aren't likely to do that, either because we haven't the ability or the interest to do so or because our schedules don't allow it. So if your goal is to lose more than just a few pounds, and you would like to lose them sooner rather than later, it makes far more sense to combine a lower-calorie diet with exercise than to rely on either exercise or diet alone to reach your goal.

What if jogging just isn't your style? Consistency and duration over the long term will also help you reach your goal. Choose an exercise you like and do it for as long as you can and as often as you can.

BOX 12

The Metabolic Equivalents (METs) of Common Activities

Activity	METs	Activity	METs
Bicycling		**Running**	
leisure	4	5 mph (12 min. mile)	8
light	6	5.2 mph	
(10–12 mph)		(11.5 min. mile)	9
moderate	8	6 mph (10 min. mile)	10
(12–14 mph)		6.7 mph (9 min. mile)	11
vigorous	10	7 mph (8.5 min. mile)	11.5
(14–16 mph)		7.5 mph (8 min. mile)	12.5
racing	12	8 mph (7.5 min. mile)	13.5
(16–19 mph)		8.6 mph (7 min. mile)	14
racing	16	9 mph (6.5 min. mile)	15
(>20 mph)		10 mph (6 min. mile)	16
		10.9 mph	
Stationary bicycling		(5.5 min. mile)	18
very light	3	cross-country	9
light	5.5	up stairs	15
moderate	7		
vigorous	10.5	**Golf**	
very vigorous	12.5	general	4.5
		carrying clubs	5.5
Circuit resistance training	8	pulling clubs	5
		using power cart	3.5
Resistance training			
light	3	**Walking**	
vigorous	6	very slow (<2.0 mph)	2
		slow (2.0 mph)	2.5
Stretching, yoga	4	slow-moderate	
		(2.5 mph)	3
Water aerobics	4	moderate (3.0 mph)	3.5
		brisk (3.5 mph)	4
Aerobics		uphill (3.5 mph)	6
general	6	very brisk (4.0 mph)	4.5
low impact	5	very, very brisk	
high impact	7	(4.5 mph)	5.0
Jogging	7		
		Walking the dog, or for	
Tennis		pleasure	3.5
general	7		
doubles	6	Walking to work or class	4
singles	8		

(cont.)

BOX 12 (cont.)

Swimming		Skiing	
freestyle laps,		general	7
(vigorous)	10	cross-country:	
freestyle laps,		light effort	7
(moderate)	8	cross-country: moderate	
backstroke laps	8	effort	8
breaststroke laps	10	cross-country: vigorous	
butterfly laps	11	effort	14
sidestroke laps	8	downhill: | light effort	5
leisurely (no laps)	6	downhill: | moderate	
Calisthenics		effort	6
vigorous	8	downhill: vigorous	
light	4.5	effort	8

Source: Adapted from B. Ainsworth et al., "Compendium of Physical Activities," *Medicine and Science in Sports and Exercise* 25 (1993): 71–80.

Believe it or not, you will be much more likely to lose weight—and keep it off—if you complete six hour-long walking sessions per week for a year than you will if you jog for 30 minutes twice a week. Why? Even though walking is a more moderate activity than jogging and burns fewer calories per minute, the total number of calories burned during the week will be greater with the six sessions of walking than the two sessions of jogging. And if you enjoy walking much more than jogging, you'll have a better chance of sticking with it.

Don't forget that regular strength training (which we discuss later in this chapter) is *essential* to weight loss. The more muscle you have, the more calories you will burn with every movement.

LEVEL 3: CARDIORESPIRATORY FITNESS

Let's say that you want to become a competent runner, cross-country skier, or bicyclist. You will need to increase the intensity of your activity from moderate to vigorous and the duration of your exercise sessions from 30 minutes to 60 minutes. You will also have to plan on training between three and five times a week to increase the strength and efficiency of your heart, lungs, and circulatory system for these activities (see Box 13).

Whatever you do, be sure to set sensible goals and start gradually so you don't get frustrated or become injured. You may also want to join a fitness center, work with a personal trainer, adopt an exercise buddy, or join an affinity group such as a running or biking club so you have people around you who support you and your goal.

Why are clear goals so important? Listen to Margot, an active 36-year-old woman who does not consider herself an athlete. One day on her way to work she saw a flood of female runners doing a 10-kilometer road race to raise money for breast cancer research and said to herself, "Next year I want to do that." As an on-again, off-again jogger, Margot had once been able to run about 3 miles. "But I knew that I had it in me to complete a longer distance—I just needed a push to get there," she said. She began planning a weekly exercise schedule that would help her get back into the jogging groove. She also joined a low-key group of runners who met at her local YMCA once a week for an extended Saturday morning run. "Some of them were really helpful in setting specific running targets, and it was great to have someone help push me farther and farther." At the end of a

BOX 13

Duration/Frequency and Intensity Required for Different Goals

Goal	Duration/Frequency	Intensity
Functional fitness/ better health/ improved mood	30 minutes or more daily	3–5 METS
Weight loss	30 to 60 minutes, 4–5 times a week	4–10 METS
Cardiorespiratory fitness	30 to 60 minutes, 3–5 times a week	5–10 METS

year, Margot entered the race and finished with a respectable time for a first-time racer.

Short-Term, Mid-Term, and Long-Term Goals

Now that you know what you want to accomplish, how do you get there? If you have been sedentary or have exercised only sporadically for most of your life, you'll need to break yourself in gently. You'll need to build up, over a matter of weeks, to 30 minutes of exercise six or seven days a week. Expecting to switch from little or no exercise to exercising *every day* is a little like expecting a car to go from 0 to 60 miles per hour in a few seconds—it can be done, but it pushes the car to its limits. Attempting to change a habit all at once isn't realistic for most people.

Let's introduce Jane here, a kind of everywoman who is a composite of many of the women we have talked with. She has two children at home, a demanding full-time job, and a husband who works long hours and travels. Consequently, Jane doesn't have a lot of extra time for exercise. Since her wedding, she has gained some weight, and now she wants it off. Ideally, she would like to lose 30 pounds in the next year. That's a tall order. At 160 pounds, Jane would have to lose nearly 20% of her weight to shed 30 pounds. Looked at that way, her goal can seem unreachable.

First off, Jane needs to break down her overall goal into more manageable chunks. What if she thought in terms of losing 2.5 pounds a month, or a bit more than one half pound a week? This is a very safe and practical rate of weight loss. Even though it adds up to 30 pounds over the course of a year, the smaller goal sounds more attainable, an important psychological strategy.

Next, let's calculate exactly how Jane could lose 2.5 pounds a month. If she takes a brisk, 30-minute walk on 24 days of a 30-day month, she would burn about 3,500 calories (150 calories × 24 days), or a pound a month. In addition, let's say she has always had a snack at night before bed. If Jane skips her late-night snack, she would save about 150 calories or more per day. Over the course of a month, this simple change would save her 4,500 calories, or just under a pound and a half, assuming she doesn't consume more calories elsewhere.

Combining these two strategies would lose Jane close to 2.5 pounds for the month. If she is consistent in her efforts over a year's time, barring any medical difficulties affecting weight loss, she will come mighty close to her goal.

If you're starting from scratch, you could resolve that your exercise goal for the first week would be to get out of bed on Tuesday, Thursday, and Saturday and walk for just 15 minutes each morning. Your goal for the first month might be to increase the length of each walking session to 30 minutes, and the frequency of those sessions to six days of the week. Sticking to these resolutions will take some effort, but you can do it.

Creating a Contract with Yourself

After setting a goal, it helps to create and write down a fairly specific plan for reaching it. Putting your thoughts in writing serves several purposes. It forces you to think through your action plan. It makes both your action plan and your goal seem real. And you can think of this written plan as a contract with yourself, something you can review whenever you need to and remind yourself of the promise you made.

First, state in writing what you intend to do overall. For Jane, this would be:

- I will burn an extra 150 calories per day by taking a brisk, 30-minute (or longer) walk each day in the morning
- I will do strength training two to three times per week
- I will skip my bedtime snack
- By the end of the first month, I will have walked 24 times and lost almost 2.5 pounds
- In a year's time, my plan is to have walked approximately 288 times and to have lost 30 pounds

Notice that achieving her long-term goal begins with small changes that gradually blossom into larger ones. A sample plan for six months might look like the one outlined in Boxes 14–17. Once you have written a similar plan of action/contract, sign it and date it and have a spouse or friend witness it to give it a more formal feeling. Ask the same person to check in with you from time to time to see how you're living up to the terms of the contract. Put your contract on your kitchen bulletin board or refrigerator, along with an easy-to-read calendar that displays the year month by month. Mark an X on the calendar each day that you walk, and each day that you make those minor adjustments in your diet. At the end of the month, you'll clearly see all the progress you've made.

BOX 14

Goals for the First Month

- **Week 1 goal: 2 days of walking; 1 day of strength training.** On Tuesday and Thursday, I will get up 45 minutes earlier and walk for 15 minutes in the morning. I will complete a 15-minute strength-training session on Wednesday morning. I will stretch for five minutes in the morning and in the evening. Diet: I will skip my evening snack.
- **Week 2 goal: 3 days of walking; 2 days of strength training.** I will walk for 15 minutes on Tuesday, Thursday, and Saturday. I will do my strength training on Wednesday and Friday. I will stretch for five minutes in the morning and in the evening. Diet: I will skip my evening snack.
- **Week 3 goal: 4 days of walking; 2 days of strength training.** I will walk for 20 minutes on Monday, Tuesday, Thursday, and Saturday, and continue strength training on Wednesday and Friday. I will stretch for five minutes in the morning and in the evening. Diet: I will skip my evening snack.
- **Week 4 goal: 5 days of walking; 2 days of strength training.** I will walk for 20 minutes Monday, Tuesday, Wednesday, Thursday, and Saturday. I will continue strength training on Wednesday and Friday. I will stretch for five minutes in the morning and in the evening. Diet: I will skip my evening snack.
- **Possible rewards:** Special flavored coffee or tea, hot bath, relaxing massage once a week.

BOX 15

Goals for the Second Month

- **Week 5 goal: 6 days of walking; 2 days of strength training.**
  I will walk 20 minutes Monday through Saturday; take Sunday
  off. I will continue strength training on Wednesday and Friday.
  I will stretch for five minutes in the morning and in the evening.
  Diet: I will skip my evening snack.
- **Week 6 goal: 6 days of walking; 2 days of strength training.**
  I will walk 25 minutes Monday through Saturday; take Sunday
  off. I will continue strength training on Wednesday and Friday.
  I will stretch for five minutes in the morning and in the evening.
  Diet: I will skip my evening snack.
- **Week 7 goal: 6 days of walking; 2 days of strength training.**
  I will walk 25 minutes Monday through Saturday; take Sunday
  off. Continue strength training on Wednesday and Friday. I will
  stretch for five minutes in the morning and in the evening. Diet:
  I will skip my evening snack.
- **Week 8 goal: 6 days of walking; 2 days of strength training.**
  I will walk 30 minutes Monday through Saturday, take Sunday
  off. I will continue strength training on Wednesday and Friday.
  I will stretch for five minutes in the morning and in the evening.
  Diet: I will skip my evening snack.
- **Possible rewards:** New walking jacket, manicure, new haircut.

Gauging Exercise Intensity

The intensity of your exercise helps determine the rate at which you burn calories. You want to find a level of activity that both meets your goal(s) and is safe.

How can you tell if your "brisk" walking pace is fast enough to give you the health benefits you're looking for? The easiest way is by monitoring your heart rate to make sure it falls into a heart rate range that is appropriate for your age.

MONITORING YOUR HEART RATE

To figure your target heart rate zone:

- subtract your age from 220
- multiply that number by 0.50 to get the lower end of the range
- multiply that number by 0.75 to get the upper end of the range

Compare this range to the chart in Box 18. For example: If you are 45 years old, you would find your range like this: 220 − 45 = 175, then

BOX 16

Goals for the Third Month—If You Wish to Go Beyond 30 Minutes a Day

- **Week 9 goal: 6 days of walking; 2 days of strength training.**
  I will walk 35 minutes Monday through Saturday, take Sunday off. I will continue strength training on Wednesday and Friday. I will stretch for five minutes in the morning and in the evening. Diet: I will skip my evening snack.
- **Week 10 goal: 6 days of walking; 2 days of strength training.**
  I will walk 40 minutes Monday through Saturday, take Sunday off. I will continue strength training on Wednesday and Friday. I will stretch for five minutes in the morning and in the evening. Diet: I will skip my evening snack.
- **Week 11 goal: 6 days of walking; 2 days of strength training.**
  I will walk 50 minutes Monday through Saturday, take Sunday off. I will continue strength training on Wednesday and Friday. I will stretch for five minutes in the morning and in the evening. Diet: I will skip my evening snack.
- **Week 12 goal: 7** days of walking; 3 days of strength training.
  I will walk 60 minutes all seven days. I will continue strength training on Wednesday and Friday. I will add a third session of strength training on Sunday. I will stretch for five minutes in the morning and in the evening. Diet: I will skip my evening snack.
- **Possible rewards:** Buy a good book or a second pair of walking shoes.

$175 \times .50 = 88$ and $175 \times .75 = 131$. That is, the safe target for your heart rate would be 88 to 131 beats per minute.

In the middle of a workout, you can measure your heart rate by placing your index and middle finger on your carotid artery—the large artery to the left or right of your voice box on your neck—or by placing them just below your wrist bone on the opposite arm. Once you feel the steady thrumming of your pulse, look at the second hand of a clock or your watch and count the number of times your heart beats within a 10-second period. Multiply that number by six to get the number of beats for one minute. If your heart is beating slower than the lowest number you calculated for your target, you will need to put a bit more effort into your workout. If it is beating faster than the highest number, ease up a bit.

If accurately tracking your time and your heart rate is important to you, think about purchasing a digital sports watch, available at many retailers for as little as $25. Even the most inexpensive models have stop-watch functions you can use to check your heart rate and track the elapsed time of your workout. The most accurate readings, though, would come from a heart rate monitor, which costs about

BOX 17

Goals for the Fourth through Sixth Months—If You Wish to Go Beyond 30 Minutes a Day

- **Weeks >12 goal: 5 days of walking; 3 days of strength training; 2 days of biking or hiking.** I will walk 60 minutes five days a week and strength train three days a week. On Saturday or Sunday, instead of walking I will substitute biking or hiking with friends and family to increase variety. I will stretch for five minutes in the morning and in the evening. Diet: I will skip my evening snack.
- **Ultimate reward:** New trail bike, new hiking boots or cross-country ski package, active vacation, membership in fitness center.

$100. Any good sporting goods store or athletic shoe dealer should be able to tell you where to get a heart rate monitor if they don't carry them.

Your target heart rate range is merely a guide, albeit a valuable one. Another easier-to-assess guide is your ability to talk while exercising. If you are unable to carry on a conversation, you are exercising too strenuously and your heart rate is probably above its safe upper limit.

As you exercise over a period of weeks, don't be surprised if the same level of activity fails to kick your heart rate up into the target

BOX 18

Target Heart Rates during Exercise

Age (years)	Target HR zone in beats per minute (50–75% of maximum)	Maximum heart rate (HR)
20	100–150	200
25	98–146	195
30	95–142	190
35	93–138	185
40	90–135	180
45	88–131	175
50	85–127	170
55	83–123	165
60	80–120	160
65	78–116	155
70	75–113	150

Source: American Heart Association

BOX 19

METs for a Day

Activity	METs	Minutes	METs X minutes
Total			

zone. As your fitness level improves, your heart will become stronger, and you'll have to increase the intensity of your activity to reach your target heart rate.

Someone who is just making the switch from a basically sedentary lifestyle should pick an activity that has a MET rating between 4 and 6. If you pick walking, this means walking at about 4 miles per hour, or a mile every 15 minutes, an activity that should be intense enough to get your heart beating between 65% to 80% of its maximum rate.

To figure out how many calories you intentionally burn in a day, fill out the "METs for a Day" table (Box 19). Multiply the total METs times minutes by your weight in pounds, then divide by 133. The result is the number of calories you used up by walking, running, climbing stairs, and so on.

Choosing Your Core Aerobic Exercise

Which exercise, or combination of exercises, is right for your daily 30-minute session? If you're not sure, take some time to think a bit about your experience with exercise, your personality, and your exercise goals. To set yourself up for success, choose the exercise that's most natural to you, and one that fits easily into your schedule. Once you've considered some of these issues, we'll help you get started— whether it's with an outdoor walking program or an indoor program that includes both aerobic exercise and strength-training exercises. The idea is to make exercise a part of your daily health maintenance routine, much as taking a shower or brushing your teeth.

Lavonne, for example, who is 38 years old, decided to get involved with different kinds of aerobic dance classes. "When I was growing up in New York City, my mom and grandmother made sure I took ballet lessons. I liked them a lot—the precision, the attention to detail, and the gracefulness all suited my needs right then. When I hit high school, I stopped, mostly because the lessons didn't give me much time for hanging out with my friends. The older I got, the less I found myself doing, physically. So when I finally decided I needed to start exercising, I tried walking and stair-stepping and some other things like that, but didn't get any enjoyment out of them. Then a girlfriend at work took me to a dance class she had been going to and I was hooked."

Taking a few minutes to fill in the answers to the questionnaire in Box 20 will help you find out more about your exercise style.

Strength Training: What's Stopping You?

In Chapter 3 we described the benefits of strength training, and in Chapters 5 and 8 we will give pointers on how to do it. But we know from talking with women about exercise that many hesitate to embark on strength training. If you fall into that camp, it may be because you have some fears or misconceptions about strength training and how it will affect your body. Let's clear those up.

MYTH: STRENGTH TRAINING RAISES BLOOD PRESSURE

That is true only for the duration of the training session. The same thing occurs with aerobic exercise. When performed properly, strength training and aerobic exercise raise systolic blood pressure (the higher of the two numbers in a blood pressure measurement) about 35 to 50 percent during the activity. Soon after exercising,

BOX 20

Your Exercise Experience and Style

1. Are there any activities you did as a child or young adult that you'd like to do again? If so, what are they?_____

_____

2. Is there any activity you've always wanted to try, but haven't made the effort to try? If so, what is it?_____

_____

3. If you don't consider yourself athletic, have you ever sensed that you might have even a little athletic ability? If so, in what area?_____

4. Is there an activity you have seen someone perform that you wanted to do yourself but were too intimidated to try? If so, what is it?_____

5. Has a friend or family member ever encouraged you to walk with him or her and you've refused? If so, why did you say no?___

_____

6. In general, do you enjoy having time to yourself, or do you prefer the company of others?_____

7. Do you prefer indoor or outdoor activities?_____

8. Do you enjoy occasional physical challenges (such as mastering a steep hill if you're walking or biking or hiking), knowing that relatively few people are able to do what you can do?_____

9. Do you prefer more social sports activities such as volleyball or tennis or racquetball, or are you more of a loner?_____

10. Would you be more comfortable being active within the social setting of a club, or at home where you can exercise at your leisure in a space you've set aside for activity?_____

blood pressure returns to its usual level. Consistent, regular strength training (or aerobic exercise), however, actually *lowers* blood pressure. For example, in a 1996 study of 785 men and women participating in a two-month program of strength and endurance exercise, systolic blood pressure dropped an average of 4 points.

Nevertheless, *if you have high blood pressure, you should talk with your doctor before beginning any exercise program.*

MYTH: STRENGTH TRAINING MAKES MUSCLES BULKY

The image that often comes to mind with strength training is the male weight lifter with bulging muscles and veins in his arms and shoulders. That's not going to happen to you, unless, of course, you want it to, and even then it would take extraordinary determination and intense effort! Women accumulate far less muscle mass than men when they engage in resistance exercise. This is mostly a function of hormones—testosterone stimulates the growth and development of muscles, and women make far, far less of this hormone than men do.

What strength training *does* do for women is tone existing muscle and build it up ever so slightly. The extra muscle is more than compensated for by the loss of fat; and since muscle is more dense than fat, meaning that ounce for ounce it takes up less space, your clothes may actually begin to fit more loosely as your muscles get stronger.

For most women, a bigger worry than gaining bulky muscles should be *losing* muscle, which always happens with age unless we do something about it. With muscle loss, you can eventually lose the ability to do simple things such as bend down and pick up something from the floor, or turn your head to see what's behind you. And far too often, muscle weakness causes a fall and a broken hip, which robs many older women of their independence.

MYTH: STRENGTH TRAINING ADDS UNWANTED WEIGHT

The key word here is unwanted. As you lose fat and gain muscle, it is likely that the scale will register an extra pound or so. But remember, that's because muscle weighs more than fat. In the long run, replacing fat with muscle increases the speed and efficiency with which your body burns calories, even at rest. Add to that the fact that you use more calories during a strength-training workout and for several hours after you've finished than you would if you were going about your daily activities, and the overall result will be an increased loss of fat and, eventually, weight.

Rather than focusing on the scale, try paying more attention to how your clothes fit. In Chapter 5 we will suggest that you measure the circumference of your waist, hips, and thighs before beginning an activity and strength-training program and then again every three months. If you walk regularly, strength train, and watch your diet as we recommend in this book, you should see some welcome changes within six months to a year.

MYTH: IF I AM SORE, I AM HURTING MYSELF

Mild soreness that appears a day or so after a workout and fades away in another day or so is actually a good sign. It means that you've stressed your muscles but they are repairing themselves and becoming stronger in the process. This stress-repair process is the key to building muscle mass.

If, of course, you experience acute pain, or a nagging pain that doesn't go away after a week, consult your doctor to make sure you haven't accidentally injured yourself. To avoid injury, we suggest that you build up the frequency, duration, and intensity of exercise gradually, to give your body time to adjust. Gentle stretching (see Chapter 8) will also help prevent injury.

MYTH: STRENGTH TRAINING AND STRETCHING TAKE TOO MUCH TIME

Only if you consider 10 to 20 minutes too much. In Chapter 8, we describe one 15-minute program and one 20-minute program for strength training. We have also included one 20-minute program that includes both strength and aerobic activity. You can cut this time in half by completing the upper body exercises in the morning and the lower body exercises at night. Or split them between two different days, if you like. Five minutes' worth of stretching should be done each morning and night, if possible.

BOX 21

Top Ten Tips for Adding Walking to a Busy Schedule

- Park your car at the farthest end of the parking lot and walk.
- Get off the subway or bus a stop early and walk a few blocks to work.
- Take a walk during your lunch break, alone or with a walking partner.
- Take the stairs rather than the elevator.
- Take your dog for a walk.
- At the mall, walk briskly around the perimeters while you window-shop.
- Instead of having a cup of coffee with a friend or colleague, get together for a walk and talk.
- Combine walking time with family time; push your children in a stroller or have them bicycle along as you walk.
- Trade child care with a neighbor so you can both have an opportunity to go outside and walk.
- Join (or start) a community or neighborhood walking club.

Finding Pockets of Time for Other Activities

- Rent an exercise tape and use it in the morning or while unwinding at night.
- Use your home exercise equipment while you're watching TV, reading, or listening to music.
- Work out with an exercise tape or home equipment while your children nap or watch a video.
- Be active with your family—shoot some baskets, go hiking, ride bikes, or throw a ball.
- Rake leaves in the fall and spend 10–15 minutes a day in the garden.
- If your workplace has a fitness room, use it regularly.
- If you travel frequently, walk in the airport while you wait and use your hotel's fitness room or swimming pool.
- Try to exercise at a regular time each day to help make it a steady habit.

Fitting It All In

Still concerned that you don't have enough room in your schedule for exercise? We suggest you use the tips in Box 21 to picture how you might fit brief bouts of walking and other exercise into your day.

Points to Remember

- Research shows that you need to burn between 1,500 and 2,000 calories per week in physical activity to attain optimum health. That benchmark can be reached by combining a daily 30-minute exercise session with activities you normally do during the course of the day and recreational activities on the weekend.
- The benefits of exercise result from a combination of how hard you exercise (intensity), how long you exercise (duration), and how often you exercise (frequency). You adjust each of these factors to achieve your particular goal.
- To make your goal possible to attain, break it down into short-term and mid-term goals that stretch you a little but are still within your reach.
- Create a plan for reaching your goal and write it down. Putting your thoughts on paper forces you to think through your plan and makes it seem real.
- Determine if you are exercising at a level of intensity that both meets your goal and is safe.
- Strength training and stretching should also be part of your regular activity program.

"Distance doesn't matter: it is only the first step that is difficult."

Marie de Vichy-Chamrond, marquise du Deffand (1697–
1780), referring to the legend that St. Denis walked
six miles carrying his head in his hand

5

Step 2: Proceed with Your Exercise Program

Now that you know more about the benefits of exercise, and how to establish an exercise habit, you're ready to measure your fitness level and establish a baseline for future reference. In this chapter, we'll ask you to take a few simple measurements and tests to determine:

- Your resting heart rate
- The time it takes for you to walk one mile
- Your strength and endurance for performing routine, daily tasks (functional capacity)
- Your fat-to-muscle ratio (gauged by your body-mass index, or BMI)
- Your waist, hip, and thigh measurements
- Your feelings about exercise

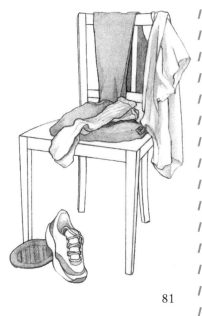

We'll ask you to record your results, along with your weight, on the "Progress Chart" in Box 22. We'll also ask you to retake these measurements and tests after 3, 6, 9, and 12 months to assess your progress. In addition,

BOX 22

Progress Chart

Test or measurement	Begin	3 months	6 months	9 months	12 months
Resting heart rate					
One-mile walking test (min)					
AHA fitness score (Box 23)					
Body Mass Index (BMI; see table)					
Waist					
Hips					
Thighs					
Weight					

we'll give you suggestions for starting an outdoor walking program and a strength-training program.

Does the term "fitness test" make you nervous or uncomfortable? Relax. You don't need to perform on this one, and you won't be graded. Better yet, only one person will see the results, and that's you. The only purpose of these tests is to identify your starting points and thus help you gauge your progress over time.

When to Check with Your Doctor

First, here's an important question you should get answered: Do you need to see your doctor before starting a walking or strength-training program?

Generally, if you are in good health, you don't have to consult your physician to begin adding a moderate amount of activity to your day, even if you have been sedentary for a while. If, however, you're planning to pursue a more vigorous program such as cycling or running, getting your doctor's blessing may be a good idea, even if you are in good health. In addition, by all means please see your doctor before starting *any* activity if any of the following is true:

- You are age 50 or older
- Your weight is 20 percent or more above your ideal body weight
- You have a family history of heart disease or stroke
- You have been diagnosed with heart disease, hypertension, type 2 diabetes, arthritis, or some other ailment

Six Simple Measurements and Tests to Assess Your Fitness Level

Take the following assessments and record the data on your "Progress Chart."

(1) RESTING HEART RATE

One key piece of physiological information is your resting heart rate, which is simply how fast your heart beats when you are *completely* at rest. All by itself, it is a fairly good measure of physical fitness—the higher your resting heart rate, the harder your heart is working and the less fit you are. Knowing your resting heart rate before you begin an exercise program will also help you see the benefits of exercise. The gradual slowing of your resting heart rate will be a kind of internal record of your progress and possibly motivate you to continue exercising.

You need to do this test before getting out of bed, because any movements you make after waking will raise your heart rate. A quick trip to the bathroom or a cup of coffee or tea will boost your heart rate well beyond its resting rate. Some morning just after you wake up and while you are still in bed, find your pulse. Place your index and middle finger on the carotid artery (the large vein to the left or right of your voice box on your neck) or an inch or so below your wrist and a bit to the outside. Move your fingers until you feel blood pulsating through the major artery below your fingers. Now turn your head ever so slightly until you can see the second hand of your watch or alarm clock and count the number of times your heart beats

BOX 23

American Heart Association Everyday Fitness Test

Aerobic Activities

1. After walking up a flight of stairs, I feel:

No discomfort   Short of breath
   1   2   3   4   5

2. After walking from gate to gate at the airport, I feel:

No discomfort   Short of breath
   1   2   3   4   5

3. After walking from one end of the mall to the other, I feel:

No discomfort   Short of breath
   1   2   3   4   5

Total points: _____

Strength Activities

4. After lifting or carrying groceries, luggage, or other heavy items, I feel:

No discomfort   Weak
   1   2   3   4   5

5. After pushing the vacuum cleaner or lawn mower, I feel:

No discomfort   Weak
   1   2   3   4   5

6. After holding a small child for several minutes, I feel:

No discomfort   Weak
   1   2   3   4   5

Total points: _____

(cont.)

BOX 23 (cont.)

Flexibility Activities

7. When bending to tie my shoes, I feel:
No discomfort   Weak
    1   2   3   4   5

8. When bending and stretching to make a bed, I feel:
No discomfort   Weak
    1   2   3   4   5

9. When reaching for the top cabinet shelf, I feel:
No discomfort   Weak
    1   2   3   4   5

Total Points: _____

Add up your total points for each of the three fitness components. If your score was between 3 and 8 for any one of the three fitness components, you're off to a good start—and you can benefit from the ideas in this book. If you scored between 9 and 15, the information we provide will help you improve your fitness level.

Source: Adapted from American Heart Association, *Fitting in Fitness* (New York: Times Books/Random House, 1997).

within a 10-second period. Multiply that number by six (for 60 seconds) to get the number of beats for one minute. Do it again, just to make sure. This is your resting heart rate. Most people have a resting heart rate between 50 and 79 beats per minute.

(2) THE ROCKPORT FITNESS WALKING TEST (ONE MILE)

Walking a mile is also a good way to gauge your fitness level. The best place to do this is on a smooth, level, one-mile stretch of road or, if you have access to it, a track at a local school or a measured walkway in a park.

- **Get ready.** Refrain from drinking caffeinated beverages or from eating a heavy meal for at least three hours before taking this test walk. Change into comfortable walking shoes and loose clothing. Take along a stopwatch or watch with a second hand and tuck a pencil and scrap of paper in your pocket.
- **Take your pulse.** Before you start walking, count your pulse for 10 seconds and multiply that number by six.
- **Warm up.** Walk a few minutes before you start.
- **Take the test.** When you are all warmed up, start your clock and walk the entire mile without stopping. Walk briskly but not so fast that you have trouble carrying on a conversation. As soon as you have finished the mile, count your pulse again for 10 seconds and multiply that number by six. Jot down this number, as well as the time it took you to walk the mile. Walk slowly for five minutes or so to cool down.
- **Check your category.** Once you have the results from your walking test, find the relative fitness chart that corresponds to your age in Boxes 24–28. Plot your time against your heart rate to determine your relative fitness level: low, high, average, above average. Do this again in 3, 6, 9, and 12 months. Record the results in your "Progress Chart."

(3) THE AMERICAN HEART ASSOCIATION EVERYDAY FITNESS TEST
While there are several ways to measure your fitness level, some of which involve seeing a physician or exercise physiologist, you can get a pretty good idea of how fit you are by reflecting upon how well you feel when you do simple, everyday tasks. The questionnaire in Box 23, developed by the American Heart Association, is intended for that purpose.

(4) YOUR BODY-MASS INDEX
It's a fact of life, and biology: tall people generally weigh more than short people. So it's impossible to set out weight guidelines that don't take height into account. Nutrition researchers have devised a single measure called body-mass index that accounts for both height and weight. You can determine yours by using the BMI chart in Box 29. Find your height in the left-hand column and read across the row to your weight. The number at the top of that column is your BMI. Re-

cord this number in your "Progress Chart." A healthy BMI is generally considered to be between 19 and 25.

If you like, you can calculate your BMI yourself by dividing your weight in pounds by your height in inches; dividing that number by your height in inches; and multiplying that number by 703.

(5) YOUR WAIST MEASUREMENT

Body type is another characteristic that can help predict your long-term health. If your body is shaped more like an apple—that is, you tend to accumulate fat around your waist and abdomen—you run a

BOX 24

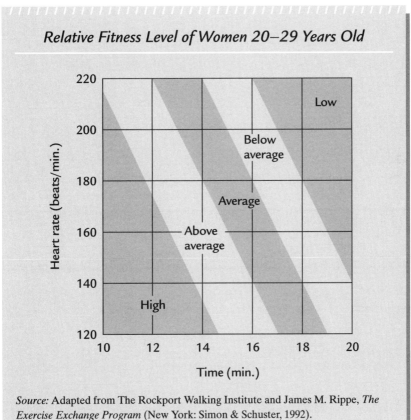

Relative Fitness Level of Women 20–29 Years Old

Source: Adapted from The Rockport Walking Institute and James M. Rippe, *The Exercise Exchange Program* (New York: Simon & Schuster, 1992).

greater risk of developing heart disease, stroke, adult-onset diabetes, high blood pressure, and some forms of cancer. On the other hand, if you are more pear-shaped—you tend to accumulate fat in your hips and thighs, rather than your waist and abdomen—your chances of developing these diseases is still higher than someone who hasn't accumulated much fat at all, but is less than those whose fat settles around the waist and abdomen.

Starting a regular activity program will help you lose fat around your middle, as well as throughout the rest of your body. Keep in

BOX 25

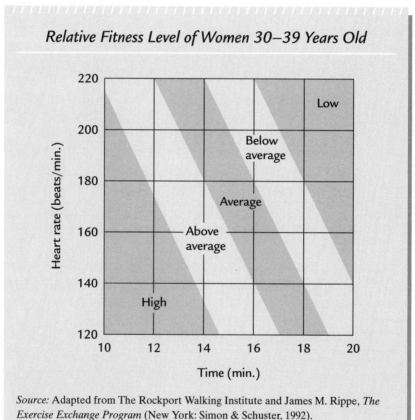

Source: Adapted from The Rockport Walking Institute and James M. Rippe, *The Exercise Exchange Program* (New York: Simon & Schuster, 1992).

mind, though, that there is no such thing as "spot reduction." You cannot lose weight in your abdomen by doing sit-ups, for example. The only way you will lose weight is by burning more calories than you take in; your body—not you—will choose which cache of stored fat to burn up first.

One good way to gauge your progress in this regard is by recording changes in your waist measurement over time. It's best to measure your waist at the narrowest part, with your stomach muscles relaxed. Record this number on your "Progress Chart."

BOX 26

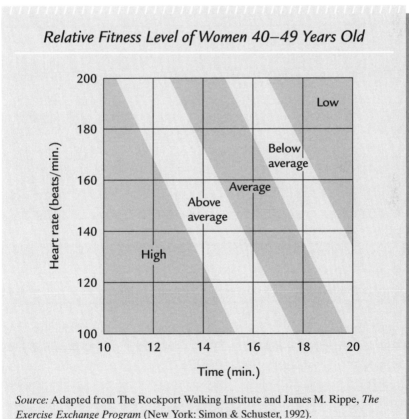

Relative Fitness Level of Women 40–49 Years Old

Source: Adapted from The Rockport Walking Institute and James M. Rippe, *The Exercise Exchange Program* (New York: Simon & Schuster, 1992).

BOX 27

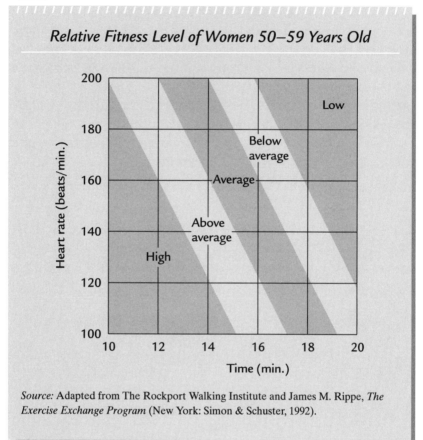

Relative Fitness Level of Women 50–59 Years Old

Source: Adapted from The Rockport Walking Institute and James M. Rippe, *The Exercise Exchange Program* (New York: Simon & Schuster, 1992).

(6) HIP AND THIGH MEASUREMENTS

Many women make the mistake of focusing on the scale as a way of marking their fitness progress. Although we've included a place on your "Progress Chart" for weight, it turns out that waist, hip, and thigh measurements are actually a much better indicator of body fat (adiposity). To measure your thighs, wrap a tape measure around each thigh where it is widest. To measure your hips, wrap a tape measure where they are widest, including the buttocks. Record these measurements on your "Progress Chart."

Your Baseline Feelings about Exercise

Now that you've taken these physical tests, we ask you to take two simple psychological tests to determine how you are feeling both physically and psychologically.

TEST 1: YOUR PERSONAL GOAL PROFILE (PGP)
This test lists some possible items that may represent your fitness goals (see Box 30). As you can see, there are spaces provided so that you can add other items that are important to you. First, decide

BOX 28

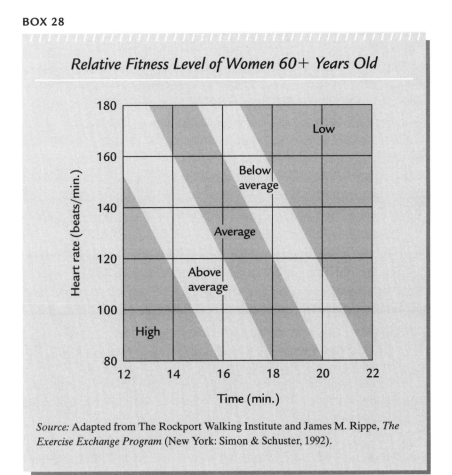

Relative Fitness Level of Women 60+ Years Old

Source: Adapted from The Rockport Walking Institute and James M. Rippe, *The Exercise Exchange Program* (New York: Simon & Schuster, 1992).

BOX 29

Body Mass Index (BMI) Table

BMI (Height)	19	20	21	22	23	24	25	26	27	28	29	30	31	32	33	34	35	36	37	38	39	40	41	42	43	44	45	46	47	48	49	50	51	52	53	54
58	91	96	100	105	110	115	119	124	129	134	138	143	148	153	158	162	167	172	177	181	186	191	196	201	205	210	215	220	224	229	234	239	244	248	253	258
59	94	99	104	109	114	119	124	128	133	138	143	148	153	158	163	168	173	178	183	188	193	198	203	208	212	217	222	227	232	237	242	247	252	257	262	267
60	97	102	107	112	118	123	128	133	138	143	148	153	158	163	168	174	179	184	189	194	199	204	209	215	220	225	230	235	240	245	250	255	261	266	271	276
61	100	106	111	116	122	127	132	137	143	148	153	158	164	169	174	180	185	190	195	201	206	211	217	222	227	232	238	243	248	254	259	264	269	275	280	285
62	104	109	115	120	126	131	136	142	147	153	158	164	169	175	180	186	191	196	202	207	213	218	224	229	235	240	246	251	256	262	267	273	278	284	289	295
63	107	113	118	124	130	135	141	146	152	158	163	169	175	180	186	191	197	203	208	214	220	225	231	237	242	248	254	259	265	270	278	282	287	293	299	304
64	110	116	122	128	134	140	145	151	157	163	169	174	180	186	192	197	204	209	215	221	227	232	238	244	250	256	262	267	273	279	285	291	296	302	308	314
65	114	120	126	132	138	144	150	156	162	168	174	180	186	192	198	204	210	216	222	228	234	240	246	252	258	264	270	276	282	288	294	300	306	312	318	324
66	118	124	130	136	142	148	155	161	167	173	179	186	192	198	204	210	216	223	229	235	241	247	253	260	266	272	278	284	291	297	303	309	315	322	328	334
67	121	127	134	140	146	153	159	166	172	178	185	191	198	204	211	217	223	230	236	242	249	255	261	268	274	280	287	293	299	306	312	319	325	331	338	344
68	125	131	138	144	151	158	164	171	177	184	190	197	203	210	216	223	230	236	243	249	256	262	269	276	282	289	295	302	308	315	322	328	335	341	348	354
69	128	135	142	149	155	162	169	176	182	189	196	203	209	216	223	230	236	243	250	257	263	270	277	284	291	297	304	311	318	324	331	338	345	351	358	365
70	132	139	146	153	160	167	174	181	188	195	202	209	216	222	229	236	243	250	257	264	271	278	285	292	299	306	313	320	327	334	341	348	355	362	369	376
71	136	143	150	157	165	172	179	186	193	200	208	215	222	229	236	243	250	257	265	272	279	286	293	301	308	315	322	329	338	343	351	358	365	372	379	386
72	140	147	154	162	169	177	184	191	199	206	213	221	228	235	242	250	258	265	272	279	287	294	302	309	316	324	331	338	346	353	361	368	375	383	390	397
73	144	151	159	166	174	182	189	197	204	212	219	227	235	242	250	257	265	272	280	288	295	302	310	318	325	333	340	348	355	363	371	378	386	393	401	408
74	148	155	163	171	179	186	194	202	210	218	225	233	241	249	256	264	272	280	287	295	303	311	319	326	334	342	350	358	365	373	381	389	396	404	412	420
75	152	160	168	176	184	192	200	208	216	224	232	240	248	256	264	272	279	287	295	303	311	319	327	335	343	351	359	367	375	383	391	399	407	415	423	431
76	156	164	172	180	189	197	205	213	221	230	238	246	254	263	271	279	287	295	304	312	320	328	336	344	353	361	369	377	385	393	402	410	418	426	435	443

To use this table, find your height (in inches) in the left-hand column. Move across to a given weight (in pounds). The number at the top of the column is your BMI.

Source: http://www.nhlbi.nih.gov/guidelines/obesity/bmi_tbl.htm

BOX 30

Personal Goal Profile (PGP)

At this moment in time:

1. Physical strength

I am far from   Goal has been
reaching my goal   attained

1 2 3 4 5 6 7 8 9 10

2. Flexibility

I am far from   Goal has been
reaching my goal   attained

1 2 3 4 5 6 7 8 9 10

3. Control of body weight

I am far from   Goal has been
reaching my goal   attained

1 2 3 4 5 6 7 8 9 10

4. Control of body fat

I am far from   Goal has been
reaching my goal   attained

1 2 3 4 5 6 7 8 9 10

5. Stress management

I am far from   Goal has been
reaching my goal   attained

1 2 3 4 5 6 7 8 9 10

6. Aerobic fitness

I am far from   Goal has been
reaching my goal   attained

1 2 3 4 5 6 7 8 9 10

7. Physical appearance

I am far from   Goal has been
reaching my goal   attained

1 2 3 4 5 6 7 8 9 10

(cont.)

BOX 30 (cont.)

8. Overall health

I am far from   Goal has been
reaching my goal   attained
1 2 3 4 5 6 7 8 9 10

9. Feeling of wellness

I am far from   Goal has been
reaching my goal   attained
1 2 3 4 5 6 7 8 9 10

10. Being physically active

I am far from   Goal has been
reaching my goal   attained
1 2 3 4 5 6 7 8 9 10

11. _____

I am far from   Goal has been
reaching my goal   attained
1 2 3 4 5 6 7 8 9 10

12. _____

I am far from   Goal has been
reaching my goal   attained
1 2 3 4 5 6 7 8 9 10

If you have other personal goals, fill them in above.

Source: Adapted from J. J. Annesi, *Enhancing Exercise Motivation* (Los Angeles: Fitness Management Books, 1996).

which items are important to you, then circle a number on the scale to indicate where you feel you are right now. The number 10 means you have fully reached that goal. You might also want to mark the items that are important to you with an asterisk (*). Disregard the items that aren't important to you. In Chapter 6, we'll ask you to take this test again after 3, 6, 9, and 12 months so you can see your progress.

TEST 2: THE EXERCISE-INDUCED FEELING INVENTORY (EFI)
While this test is most often used to determine how an individual feels right after an exercise session, we ask you to take this simple test right now to determine how, in general, you feel about your current lifestyle (see Box 31). The idea is to repeat it later after exercise

BOX 31

Exercise-Induced Feeling Inventory (EFI)

At this moment in time, I feel:

1. Refreshed
Do not feel   Feel very strongly
1 2 3 4 5 6 7 8 9 10

2. Calm
Do not feel   Feel very strongly
1 2 3 4 5 6 7 8 9 10

3. Fatigued
Do not feel   Feel very strongly
1 2 3 4 5 6 7 8 9 10

4. Enthusiastic
Do not feel   Feel very strongly
1 2 3 4 5 6 7 8 9 10

5. Relaxed
Do not feel   Feel very strongly
1 2 3 4 5 6 7 8 9 10

6. Energetic
Do not feel   Feel very strongly
1 2 3 4 5 6 7 8 9 10

7. Happy
Do not feel   Feel very strongly
1 2 3 4 5 6 7 8 9 10

(cont.)

BOX 31 (cont.)

8. Tired

Do not feel   Feel very strongly

1 2 3 4 5 6 7 8 9 10

9. Revived

Do not feel   Feel very strongly

1 2 3 4 5 6 7 8 9 10

10. Peaceful

Do not feel   Feel very strongly

1 2 3 4 5 6 7 8 9 10

11. Worn-out

Do not feel   Feel very strongly

1 2 3 4 5 6 7 8 9 10

12. Upbeat

Do not feel   Feel very strongly

1 2 3 4 5 6 7 8 9 10

The idea is to focus your attention on: positive engagement (items 4, 7, 12); revitalization (items 1, 6, 9); tranquility (items 2, 5, 10); and physical exhaustion (items 3, 8, 11).

Source: Adapted from L. Gauvin and W. J. Rejeski, "The Exercise-Induced Feeling Inventory: Development and Initial Validation," *Journal of Sport and Exercise Psychology* 15, no. 4 (1993): 409.

sessions to make you aware of how your feelings change—and if you are exercising at an appropriate intensity level. Obviously, if you feel calm, refreshed, happy, enthusiastic, or relaxed after exercising, your program is enhancing your lifestyle. On the other hand, if you feel fatigued, tired, or worn out, you might be overdoing it. In that case, try shortening your workout a bit and make sure you're getting enough sleep and eating a balanced, nutritious diet.

Starting a Walking Program

Let's say you have chosen walking as your activity for many of the reasons we've mentioned, as well as for some of your own. Your daily program might be the one for beginners suggested by the American Heart Association (see Box 32). You'd like to start walking on Monday morning. To prepare, do the following sometime during the preceding week, and definitely before Sunday afternoon.

BOX 32

Walking Program for Beginners

Week	Exercise	Warm up + exercise + cool down
1	Walk briskly 5 min.	15 min.
2	Walk briskly 7 min.	17 min.
3	Walk briskly 9 min.	19 min.
4	Walk briskly 11 min.	21 min.
5	Walk briskly 13 min.	23 min.
6	Walk briskly 15 min.	25 min.
7	Walk briskly 18 min.	28 min.
8	Walk briskly 20 min.	30 min.
9	Walk briskly 23 min.	33 min.
10	Walk briskly 26 min.	36 min.
11	Walk briskly 28 min.	38 min.
12	Walk briskly 30 min.	40 min.

Source: American Heart Association

- **Mark a good, safe course:** Use your car's odometer to find an appropriate one-mile route that you can traverse safely any time of the day. Or look for a track at a local high school that will be safe to use. At the same time, you might also scope out an indoor location such as a local mall or even an airport that you can use when it is extremely hot or raining or snowing heavily. Because safety is an important concern for women, we've included a list of safety tips based on recommendations from the Road Runners Club of America (see Box 33). In a few weeks, when you've progressed, you may want to add an additional mile onto that course if you can, with a challenging hill if there's one available.

- **If you haven't done so, take the Rockport Walking Test in this chapter and record your results:** It shouldn't take you much more than 15 minutes to complete the test, and doing so will give you a starting point you can use to gauge your progress over the next few weeks and months.

- **If you haven't done so, set short-term, mid-term, and long-term goals:** As part of forming an exercise habit, you'll need to break down your large goal—improved health, endurance, or weight loss—into smaller, more manageable goals (see Chapter 4). Accomplishing these smaller goals will give you a sense of mastery. If you can stick with exercise long enough to feel these positive feelings, you'll be well on your way toward making exercise an important part of your life.

- **Buy a pair of good, comfortable walking shoes:** Walking shoes should have enough cushion to absorb the impact of each step and enough room to allow for a pair of cotton sports socks.

- **Select loose, comfortable clothing that's suited to the weather:** On a hot, humid summer day, wear breathable cotton, or a cotton-and-Lycra blend and try to exercise early in the morning, or later in the afternoon or evening. If it's cold, dress in layers, starting with a T-shirt or two next to your skin, followed by a turtleneck and a windbreaker. If it's windy, consider wearing a pair of cotton-and-Spandex leggings underneath nylon pants. And don't forget to protect your head and hands with a hat and gloves, and wear a scarf. Once you warm up, you can remove the gloves or the hat to cool off. A little experimentation with layers will show you the right mix of clothing for your comfort level on a particular day.

BOX 33

Safety Tips for Walking and Running

- Don't wear headphones. Use your ears to be aware of your surroundings.
- Run or walk with a partner or a dog.
- Carry some change in case you need to make a phone call.
- Write down or leave word of where you are headed. Tell friends and family of your favorite routes.
- Stick to familiar areas. (If you're new to an area, contact a local Road Runners Club of America or running store.) Know where telephones are, or open businesses or stores.
- Alter your route.
- Stay alert. The more aware you are, the less vulnerable you are.
- Avoid unpopulated areas, deserted streets, and overgrown trails. Especially avoid unlit areas at night. Steer clear of parked cars or bushes.
- Carry identification or write your name, phone number, and blood type on the inside sole of your shoe. Include any medical information. Don't wear jewelry.
- Ignore verbal harassment. Use discretion in acknowledging strangers. Look directly at others and be observant, but keep your distance and keep moving.
- Run or walk against traffic so you can observe approaching automobiles.
- Wear reflective material if you choose to exercise before dawn or after dark.
- Use your intuition about a person or an area. If you're unsure, go with your gut instinct.
- Practice memorizing license tags or identifying characteristics of strangers.
- Carry a noisemaker or whistle.
- Call police immediately if something happens to you or someone else, or you notice anyone out of the ordinary.

As a rule, you'll probably be surprised how little clothing you'll need even when it's cold. Your body can generate an enormous amount of heat during a brisk walk. And finally, keep in mind that if you wait for perfect weather, chances are you won't be able to walk regularly. You may have to walk when it's raining a bit; but as you warm up, you might come to appreciate a little drizzle on your face. Besides, learning to walk in a light rain can help you enjoy days that other people are likely to find a little depressing.

DAY ONE AND WEEK ONE

If you really want to be successful, please take this advice:

- **Make things as easy on yourself as you can:** The night before you plan to start exercising, put your jacket, shoes, and any other gear out in plain view near the back door—or near your bed. Some women even wear their exercise T-shirt and sweatpants to bed the night before, so they're all dressed for exercise the minute they wake up.
- **Drink enough fluid:** Whatever the weather, it's a good idea to drink a glass or two of water before you walk to keep your body properly hydrated. Whether you realize it or not, you're going to sweat even on a cool day. Adequate hydration, of course, is very important on a very hot and humid day. Take a plastic water bottle with you and drink from it frequently to prevent heat stress.
- **Warm up:** As you start, walk slowly for a few minutes to allow your muscles to warm up and loosen up. This will help prevent injury.
- **Use good walking technique:** While it's true that walking is a natural activity, there are some things you can do to get the most from your walking session. Consider the five tips for better walking technique suggested by the editors of *Walking Magazine* (Box 34).
- **Take five minutes to cool down:** The idea here is to walk slowly to allow your heart rate to slow down. An adequate cool-down period will also help to prevent muscle soreness. It's also a good idea to do your daily stretching shortly after you've walked—while your muscles are still warm.

- **Find support, if you need it:** If starting a walking program on your own seems too difficult, you may want to join a walking group. Some YMCAs and private health clubs have begun "exercise outreach programs" designed to appeal to people in their communities who want to start exercising but need a little encouragement to get started.
- **Break yourself in gently:** Tell yourself that your goal for that very first morning is to get out of bed, put on your jacket and walking shoes, and go out the door to walk for 15 minutes or so. Don't necessarily expect to do that *every* morning of the first week. Plan on two or three times a week—say on Tuesday and Thursday, or Monday, Wednesday, and Friday. If possible, have someone else in your household get up with you. If you can't conceive of exercising before your usual morning routine, scan the paper while you have your coffee or tea and *then* go.
- **Record and reward your progress:** It is very important to give yourself credit for any exercise you do. Write down what you did, how you feel about your accomplishment, and reward yourself for doing it. Recording this information will give it validity; rewarding it will reinforce positive feelings associated with it. The appropriate logs are supplied for you in Chapters 6 and 7.

BOX 34

Five Tips for Better Walking Technique

- Walk tall, lifting your chest and shoulders.
- Gently contract your stomach muscles to flatten your lower back.
- To go faster, concentrate on quick steps instead of long ones.
- Land on your heel and roll your foot from heel to toe, pushing off forcefully with your toes.
- For a speed boost, bend your elbows to 90°; swing your hands from your waistband to chest height.

Starting a Strength-Training Program

Strength training conditions your heart, improves your muscular endurance, and strengthens your tendons and ligaments. In general, it also helps to increase muscle mass and stimulates bone growth.

While there are several types of strength training, we are assuming you will initially be exercising at home, so we will discuss *dynamic constant-resistance exercise,* which you can do with your own body weight (push-ups, sit-ups, pull-ups) or with free weights. The term "resistance" refers to the fact that when you lift your body or a free weight, you exert a certain amount of force to work against gravity. Doing this on a consistent basis strengthens your muscles.

The other form—*dynamic variable-resistance exercise*—requires exercise equipment with levers, cams, or linkage systems that automatically increase the resistance. You're not likely to have this kind of strength-training equipment at home.

Strength training stimulates muscle growth. Your muscles respond to increased stress by developing larger fibers. Larger muscle fibers lead to larger muscles (but not too large in women), which have greater strength and take more energy to maintain. Without such stimulus, muscles atrophy—their cells degenerate. If you or someone close to you has ever broken an arm or leg bone and worn a cast for a number of weeks, you've seen a rather dramatic form of atrophy. Take the cast off of a broken leg, compare it to a healthy leg, and you'll see that the muscles have shrunk and will build up again only with regular use. The atrophied leg is an obvious example of the type of degeneration that occurs to your muscles over decades—if you do not strength train.

How much strength training do you need? Once again, the answer depends on your goals. If you want to maintain muscle for functional fitness—you want to stay strong enough to carry your own suitcases at the airport, or to lug a couple of heavy bags of groceries—two workouts a week (with 24 to 48 hours in between to allow for muscle repair and growth) should be adequate. At this level, depending on your weight and body type, you may see some toning effect within a few months, proving your workouts are consistent.

In terms of adding muscle and losing fat, two workouts per week is almost as good as three. In a study done by Wayne Westcott, the

Massachusetts strength-training researcher we met earlier, more than a thousand men and women started doing 25 minutes of strength training on Nautilus machines plus 15 to 20 minutes of walking on a treadmill or cycling on a stationary cycle. Those who trained twice a week added an average of two pounds of muscle and lost four pounds of fat, while those who trained three times a week added 2.5 pounds of muscle and lost 4.5 pounds of fat. Clearly, three workouts a week yield greater benefits than two, but not significantly greater benefits.

Planning for three workouts per week, though, isn't a bad strategy. "If you strive for three and miss one, you've still done two. If you strive for two and miss one, then you may be headed for trouble," says Westcott. One workout per week offers nowhere near the benefits of two and may leave you open to injury.

If you are aiming for more than functional fitness and want to add more muscle mass and tone for appearance's sake, or to improve your performance in a particular sport, then we suggest that you consult a personal trainer, a strength-training video, or a book for a specific program to meet your needs. Seeking advice will also ensure that you learn good strength-training form and technique.

What Does Mild Muscle Soreness Mean?

Strengthening your muscles means challenging them with increasing amounts of physical stress (exercise). You must work them until they tire, give them a chance to rest and rebuild, then stress them again, gradually increasing the amount of stress. The more stress your muscles experience—within reason—the stronger they become. What is actually happening inside the muscle tissue is that you are creating small tears in the muscle fibers. The repair process not only fixes the tears but makes new muscle in that region as well.

You won't create the necessary muscle strain unless you lift 75% of the maximum you are able to lift—a safe level for most people. If you can complete between 8 and 12 controlled repetitions of a particular exercise before your muscle fatigues, then you should be at 75% of your maximum. *Controlled repetitions* means you complete each set of 8 to 12 in 50 to 70 seconds.

You will know muscle fatigue when you see it or feel it. The affected muscle temporarily loses its ability to lift or pull and may begin to shake a bit. Remember, a small amount of muscle fatigue is necessary and temporary, and it's a signal that the muscle is being appropriately challenged.

If strength training is new to you, and you have properly exercised your muscles to the point of fatigue, you will probably experience mild muscle soreness a day or so after your exercise session. This mild soreness is actually a good sign, indicating that you have stressed the muscle enough. With a day or two of rest, the muscle will repair and rebuild itself to greater strength. That is why you should not strength train the same group of muscles more than three times per week, with a 36- to 48-hour break in between each session. As the weeks go by and your muscles become stronger, you will need to add even more resistance (weight) to stress them even further.

In Chapter 8 we will present in detail three programs that will get you started with strength training on a couple of days each week, as well as a set of stretching exercises that you ought to perform every day.

Points to Remember

- The tests in this chapter can help you determine how fit you are now so you can observe how much progress you make from this point onward.
- Be sure to follow the suggestions given for starting your walking program. They will ensure that you get started "on the right foot" and progress at a healthy, natural pace.
- As you begin to strength train, keep in mind that some discomfort in the form of mild muscle soreness is to be expected. It is just an indication that you are working your muscles hard enough to strengthen them. Any soreness you feel should disappear in a few days as your muscles rebuild themselves.
- To protect yourself from injury, be sure to complete the stretching exercises described in Chapter 8. For best results, spend 5 minutes stretching every morning and 5 minutes every evening. You'll find that it's a great way to prepare yourself for your day and to unwind at night.

> "I write entirely to find out what I'm thinking, what I'm looking at, what I see and what it means, what I want, and what I fear."
>
> Joan Didion (1934–), essayist and novelist

6

Step 3:
Record Your Progress

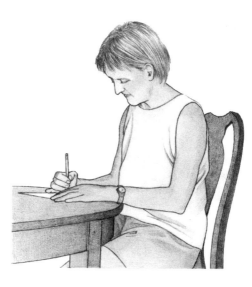

In this chapter, we'll ask you to retake the "Personal Goal Profile" (PCP) and the "Exercise-Induced Feeling Inventory" (EFI) from Chapter 5, as well as the "Lifestyle Inventory" and "Mind/Body Inventory" from Chapter 1, to focus your attention on your feelings. We also strongly suggest that you record your physical activity on the logs provided in Boxes 35 and 36 so that you can monitor your own efforts. And because the first three months of an exercise program can be a challenge, we offer some suggestions as to what you might expect to experience during that important initial phase.

BOX 35

Walking Log

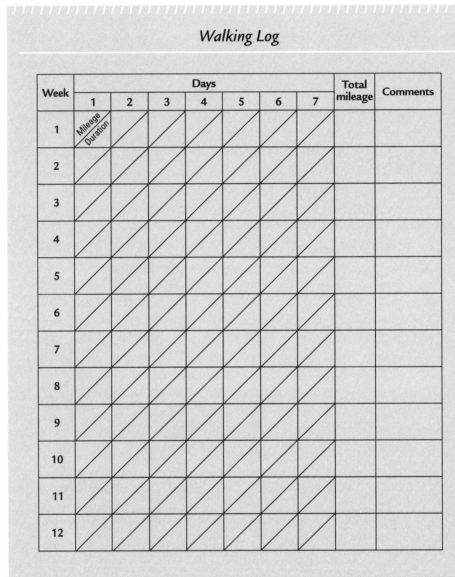

Week	Days							Total mileage	Comments
	1	2	3	4	5	6	7		
1	Mileage / Duration								
2									
3									
4									
5									
6									
7									
8									
9									
10									
11									
12									

BOX 36

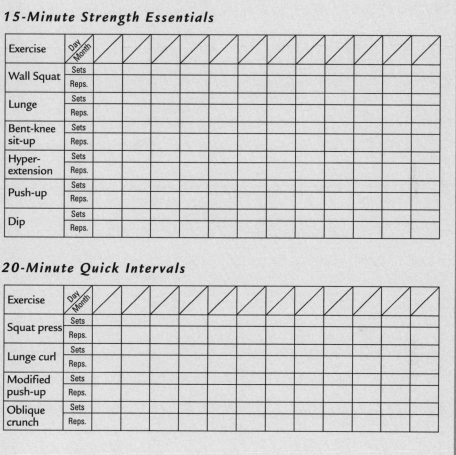

Strength-Training Logs

15-Minute Strength Essentials

Exercise	Day/Month												
Wall Squat	Sets												
	Reps.												
Lunge	Sets												
	Reps.												
Bent-knee sit-up	Sets												
	Reps.												
Hyper-extension	Sets												
	Reps.												
Push-up	Sets												
	Reps.												
Dip	Sets												
	Reps.												

20-Minute Quick Intervals

Exercise	Day/Month												
Squat press	Sets												
	Reps.												
Lunge curl	Sets												
	Reps.												
Modified push-up	Sets												
	Reps.												
Oblique crunch	Sets												
	Reps.												

A major goal of this chapter is to focus your attention on the positive changes you will experience within the first few weeks of your new exercise program. Those changes will be largely *psychological*— stress reduction, mood elevation, an increase in energy, a feeling of vitality, a sense of pride from your accomplishment. These mainly stem from exercise's mild "addictive effect," the result of changes in

BOX 36 (cont.)

20-Minute Total Body Basics

Exercise	Day/Month	/	/	/	/	/	/	/	/	/	/	/
Dumbbell Squat	Sets											
	Reps.											
Step-up	Sets											
	Reps.											
Calf raise	Sets											
	Reps.											
Bent-over row	Sets											
	Reps.											
Back fly	Sets											
	Reps.											
Barbell curl	Sets											
	Reps.											
Tricep extension	Sets											
	Reps.											
Chest press	Sets											
	Reps.											
Chest fly	Sets											
	Reps.											
Shoulder Press	Sets											
	Reps.											
Upright row	Sets											
	Reps.											
Crunch	Sets											
	Reps.											
Hyper-extension	Sets											
	Reps.											

your brain chemistry that relax you and relieve pain. Once you experience these feelings, you'll want more of them.

However, because most of us think of exercise results in terms of *physiological* changes such as weight loss and toning, we tend to underestimate—or worse, completely ignore—the positive feelings that exercise induces. We want those changes everyone can see, and we want them fast. If your expectations are dominated by hopes of such rapid physical changes, you're likely to become discouraged and feel like quitting.

The best way to build an exercise habit is to concentrate on changes in your emotional well-being and to relax as you give your body time to change. Positive feelings will help you form an exercise habit that, in time, will result in desirable changes in your physical being. Once those physiological changes start to happen—improvements in blood pressure, cholesterol levels, and blood sugar can appear within several weeks—they will serve to reinforce your exercise habit even further.

Recording Your Activity

One of your major goals should be to increase the overall level of activity in your day, some of which is exercise. Remember the "fidget factor" study? Its main message was that everything active you do in a day counts toward keeping you trimmer and healthier. So it's a good idea to record every now and then exactly what you did during the day as a way to make yourself aware of how active you really are. Use the walking and strength-training logs provided in Boxes 35 and 36.

What Should You Expect in the First 12 Weeks?

Beginning exercisers experience many new feelings, and also face many new challenges, during the first critically important weeks of an exercise program. These may be much easier to handle if you know they are common to many women like you. So we've gathered some of the more common reactions, based on James Annesi's years of research in health clubs across the country.

WEEKS 1–4

During the first few weeks of an exercise program, it is not unusual to feel a little intimidated by the thought of exercise, and maybe a bit alone. If you don't feel this way, that's wonderful. If you do, we suggest that you dress in exercise clothing that you're completely comfortable wearing, find a partner with whom you can exercise, and focus your mind down the road a few weeks. Exercise will feel more natural each time you do it.

It's very important to start your program gradually. If you've never exercised before, it's too much to expect that you'll immediately start exercising six or seven days a week. In addition, set some short-term, mid-term, and long-term goals in the form of a written contract with yourself if you haven't already done so, just to clarify what you intend to do and how often. Chapter 4 covers the basics of goal-setting.

Retaking the "Personal Goal Profile" (Box 30) and the "Exercise-Induced Feeling Inventory" (Box 31) is especially important in this early phase. Doing so puts you in touch with positive perceptual changes ("I have more energy," or "I *feel* thinner") that come long before changes in physiology.

The "Personal Goal Profile" will show you how you are progressing toward your goals. Be sure to retake it at the end of week four. The "Exercise-Induced Feeling Inventory" is most often used to determine how an individual feels right after an exercise session, so you'll want to repeat this test after your exercise sessions to make you aware of how your feelings change—and if you are exercising at an appropriate intensity level. If you feel calm, refreshed, happy, enthusiastic, or relaxed, exercise is enhancing your lifestyle. On the other hand, if you feel fatigued, tired, or worn out, you're probably overdoing it. In that case, try shortening your workout a bit and make sure you're getting enough sleep and eating a balanced, nutritious diet. If your start has been a little sporadic, make consistency your goal for next month.

WEEKS 5–8

By this time, your "Exercise Balance Sheet" may be shifting more toward the positive. If you haven't filled one out, go ahead and do one. You'll find that it helps authenticate this shift (see Box 37).

Here's a reality check: If you've chosen to walk 30 minutes a day and have not severely restricted your calorie intake (which we do not suggest you do), you probably won't have lost more than a pound or two, if that. In fact, if you have been strength training, you may have gained a little weight. *This is a good sign;* it means that you are adding muscle. You may also want to take the "Personal Goal Profile" once more to reinforce any growing positive feelings you have begun to experience. At least look at the calendar (or the log in this chap-

BOX 37

Exercise Balance Sheet

Activity	Time frame	Negatives	Positives

ter) you have used to record your workouts and take pride in the fact the you've come this far.

WEEKS 9–12

Congratulations! Chances are you're into a well-established routine by now. But is that a problem? Are you getting a little bored? If so, try something new. Get a portable CD player, tape player, or radio so you can listen to music or to a book-on-tape during your walk. Follow a new exercise route or do your usual route in reverse. Join a walking or hiking group. Or maybe a new indoor activity like cycling would complement your outdoor walking program nicely. Try anything you can think of—even new exercise togs—to keep it interesting.

We also encourage you to retake the six tests and measurements that you took in Chapter 5 to assess your fitness level—now, after 3 months, and again at the 6-, 9-, and 12-month marks—and record the results in your "Progress Chart." These were:

- Your resting heart rate
- The AHA Everyday Fitness Test
- The Rockport Fitness Walking Test
- Your body-mass index
- Your waist measurement
- Your hip and thigh measurements

At first, you will undoubtedly note changes in some areas and not others. The key is not to expect too much of your body. Simply know that you are improving your overall health and give your body time to adapt to your new regimen.

Points to Remember

- For the first few months of exercise, be sure to focus on the positive feelings that exercise induces. Physiological changes will come later.
- Each time you exercise, record your activity on a calendar or one of the logs we provide so you can observe your own progress.
- Be sure to retake the other physical fitness tests from Chapter 5 so you can monitor changes in your physiology and functional fitness.

"The ultimate of being successful is the luxury of giving yourself the time to do what you want to do."

Leontyne Price (1927–), opera singer

7

Step 4:
Reward Your Efforts

We've included reward as the last part of our four-step plan because appropriate rewards have tremendous power to reinforce behavior. We're not only creatures of habit, we are creatures of pleasure as well, as this passage from *Healthy Pleasures* by Robert Ornstein, Ph.D., and David Sobel, M.D., makes abundantly clear:

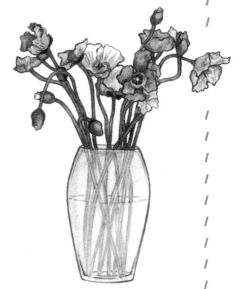

Imagine the world without pleasure. Life would appear colorless and humorless. A baby's smile would go unappreciated. Foods would be tasteless. The beauty of a Bach concerto would fall on deaf ears. Feelings like joy, thrills, delights, ecstasy, elation, and happiness would disappear. The company of others would not bring comfort and joy. The touch of a mother would not soothe, and a lover could not arouse. Interest in sex and procreation would dry up. The next generation would go unborn.

Fortunately, life is not like that. Nerve pathways speed satisfying sensations to the brain. Packets of chemicals stand ready to transmit

113

pleasure signals from one nerve cell to another. There is a pleasure machine within our head, in which several brain centers respond to gratifying stimulation.

All this didn't happen by accident; the human desire for enjoyment evolved to enhance our survival. What better way to assure that healthy, life-saving behaviors occur than to make them pleasurable?

While we encourage you to exercise for your health, we want to remind you to exercise for pleasure. If you must get up at dawn to walk, notice the quiet, the peace, and the slight pink tint to the sky when you walk out the back door. Smell the freshness in the air. Breathe deeply as you walk, and notice how the air both wakes you up and helps you to relax at the same time. Or if you walk at lunch time, enjoy the break from too much work and too many interruptions and remind yourself how much better you feel all afternoon on days when you've taken a lunchtime walk. Appreciate these moments in your day, whenever you can.

One way to keep you connected with your chosen activity is to attach to it some meaningful rewards. That way, instead of thinking of exercise as yet another task on an endless list of chores, or as time away from something else you'd rather be doing—such as sleeping— we'd like to help you condition yourself to make *positive associations* with physical activity. In a world that puts too many demands on your time, emotions, and energy, it would be wonderful if you could think of your exercise session as a precious opportunity to invest these assets in yourself. You, who do so much for others, sometimes need to do for yourself.

Laura, who is 56, has created an exercise habit around a *reward*— her favorite hobby, listening to books on tape. "On a weekend morning, I put on my exercise clothes as soon as I get up. I also put a tape into my Walkman and put it in the pocket of my sweatpants. Then, I listen to the book as I'm folding the laundry, doing the dishes, or other chores. I find that I get so involved with the tape, that it's easy for me to just go out the door and start walking."

Some people make mistakes with rewards, choosing activities that make them feel good for a moment but a bit guilty soon afterward. If you're on a tight budget, would buying yourself a new dress really make you feel good, or would you regret spending that money? If weight loss is a goal of your exercise program, would the extra calories of an ice cream cone really make you feel good, or would you regret it after the last bite? Of course, if an ice cream cone or a new dress really does make you feel good, go for it! We're not suggesting that you feel guilty about such treats, only that you choose a reward that enhances, rather than detracts from, your emotional well-being.

Here are some suggested rewards:

- **Small:** An extra hour of sleep on Saturday, brunch on Sunday, fresh flowers from the florist, new earrings, your favorite bottle of cologne, a new CD to play as you walk (or whatever makes you feel great)
- **Medium:** New workout clothes, a dress you've been eyeing for a special occasion, a course in yoga to help you relax, a pair of tickets for the symphony (or whatever makes you feel great)
- **Large:** Trading in your old car for a newer one, hiring a professional landscaper to redesign your backyard, taking a quick trip to Paris for no reason (or whatever makes you feel great)

Staying with It—When It's Not Easy

We've been encouraging you to build your exercise habit slowly and consistently. At the same time, we fully recognize that exercising on some days will be harder than others, probably because something in your life is out of balance—perhaps you've had too little to eat, too little sleep, too much stress at home or at the job. The variables are numerous. We've tried to anticipate a few of them and offer suggestions on how to surmount them.

- **You're too tired, or you'd rather eat than exercise:** Poor eating or sleeping habits can greatly affect your motivation to exercise. If it's 6 a.m. or 6 p.m., and you feel too tired to walk, it could be that you just need a light snack to perk you up. Don't eat too much, though, because a heavy meal is likely to make you feel more sluggish. You want to strike a balance. And make sure you get enough sleep. Good food and adequate sleep will help you feel more positive about your activity program—and about everything else you need to accomplish during your day.

- **It doesn't feel right:** Most of us are very resistant to change. But give yourself time—a month at least—to adjust. One mistake people often make is giving up before they can experience the pleasure of exercise—a feeling of accomplishment, more restful sleep, improved muscle tone, and, depending on your particular situation, the companionship of a friend or family member who exercises with you. At the same time, don't be surprised if, on certain days, that hill in the middle of your walk is an unusual challenge. Even when you're in good shape, your routine may, on occasion, take a little extra effort to complete because you're stiff, you haven't been eating properly, you're overly tired, or you've just recovered from the flu. Accept the fact that you're going to have "off days." When this occurs, the best thing to do is just get it done and be proud of yourself that you did.

- **You don't feel up to it:** Our best advice: Get moving anyway—unless you have a fever, bad cold, or some other illness. If you're feeling tired, tell yourself you're going to do half of your normal workout. There's a very good chance that, once you start, you'll feel more energized and complete the whole thing. Of course, if you've had a prolonged illness, check with your doctor before resuming your activity program. But if you have to stop for a day or two because of a cold, or a week because of the flu, you should be able to get right back into your program. If you're off for a week, try walking 20 minutes instead of 30 minutes your first day back. Listen to your body—it will let you know how much exercise it can handle.

- **Your exercise partner can't make it:** It's wonderful to walk with a spouse or partner. Chances are, you get involved in a conversation and your workout is over before you know it. But don't let yourself depend too much on someone else or their schedule. If you do, you probably will find it difficult to exercise regularly. When your partner is absent, get out and walk anyway. Try bringing a small radio or cassette-player to keep you company.

- **You're depressed:** While exercise may be the last thing you feel like doing right now, *it is probably the one thing you need to do the most.* If facing your regular workout is just too much on a given day, cut it in half, or even a third. Put on your comfortable exercise clothes, try some stretching exercises, and breathe deeply. If you can make yourself get started and exercise long enough for the endorphins to kick in, there's a good chance you'll finish your workout. And you'll be grateful, really grateful, that you've discovered exercise as a way of successfully coping with dark moods. Whatever problem you're battling, exercise can help you put it in perspective.

Remember 59-year old Mary from Chapter 3? Over time, she has learned to exercise (she walks on her indoor treadmill) even when she's not in the mood. "I do say to myself, 'When the going gets tough, the tough get going.' And it helps. I had a day the other day when I just didn't know if I could finish, but I did. It was just hard. I do know that every time is different. Sometimes I don't feel like exercising in the beginning, but then I move into it. I've told myself I'll do half, and then I find that I've finished. I just put one foot in front of the other."

What Is a Relapse?

It's inevitable, is what it is. Life gets in the way. On some days you simply won't be able to take your walk. And at some points in your life, one day off will drift into two, then three. Before you know it, an entire week has gone by. If you've had the flu or some other nasty illness for a week or so, it may take you as long as another week to get back to your routine. The same kind of thing can happen when your daily routine changes—you take a new job, move to a new home, or have a sick child, spouse, or parent who needs your attention. Sometimes out-of-town visitors upset your schedule, or travel plans get in the way.

When this inevitably occurs, you'll need to reassess your schedule and reconfigure your goals. If you have been away from exercise for two weeks or more, don't expect to complete your usual workout. Cut the time in half the first few days you're back in order to give your body—and your mind—time to readjust.

One secret to exercise success is to keep your confidence when you relapse. Don't judge yourself harshly if you've missed some exercise sessions. That's a waste of emotional energy. Instead, invest that energy into getting started again. While it's important to take your exercise training very seriously, it's also important to remember that missing a day or two, or even a week or two, here and there doesn't really matter in the big picture of your health and well-being. The important thing is to get out the door and get started once again.

Of course, this is easier said than done. It may be hard to get restarted because, during your relapse, you may have slipped backward from the "action" or "maintenance" stage of change to the "preparation" or even "contemplation" stage (see Chapter 3). If you've had a relapse of a week, two weeks, or even longer, the notion of exercising can once again feel foreign—almost as if you had never formed a habit in the first place.

The good news—no, the *great* news—is that it can take you as little as one workout, or even a session that's half as long as a normal session, to get you back in the spirit again. So if you relapse, take it one day at a time. Tell yourself, "I'm going to work out only half as long today, just to get myself to do it. I'll worry about tomorrow when tomorrow comes." Chances are, once you get into your exercise clothes, out the door, and down the block, your workout will seem so natural that you'll feel as if you never stopped.

If you relapse, we suggest you do what Mary does—take missed workouts in stride, and focus on restarting your workouts as soon as you can. "I don't make myself feel guilty if I miss a workout," says Mary. "I have a commitment that I will get to it tomorrow. Now I am very interested in exercising four or five times per week. I'll make sure I do it on Saturday and Sunday, because it's during the week that I get into trouble—when I don't have enough time."

Tools You Can Use to Get Back on Track

If you get out of your walking habit and have a tough time getting back to it, try using some of the mental exercises below to give yourself a jumpstart:

- **Mental imagery or visualization:** For some people, mental "rehearsals" are a helpful tool for converting a wish into action. Mental imagery and visualization basically work like this: Sit and relax for a few minutes. Close your eyes and imagine yourself exercising. Don't spare any details. Picture yourself putting on your walking shoes, grabbing your keys, opening and closing the front door, striding down your front walk, and out into the sidewalk. Try to conjure up the sound of the early birds, if you're a morning walker, or the closing hush of the day if you're more partial to evening exercise. Feel the wind in your face, the spring in your feet as you walk past familiar checkpoints. Capture in your imagination, if you can, the things that you enjoy most about exercising. Sometimes an armchair walk or two can help you do the real thing again.

- **Positive reinforcement:** All along, you've been writing down what you have accomplished and rewarding yourself for accomplishing it. On a tough day, review your exercise logs and think of an appealing reward at the end of your walk.

- **Rehearsal and stimulus control:** Put things into your environment to remind you of exercise and prepare yourself so it's easy for you to go for a walk or a workout. Call up a friend and make a date for the next day's walk. Hang your walking jacket on the back door, with your walking shoes nearby. Maybe even wear your exercise clothes to bed the night before!

- **Supportive set-ups:** Get on the phone and gather a group of three friends to walk with you for three out of the six to seven days you walk. Take your walks to pretty settings such as a local arboretum or river walk. Take your dogs with you to walk around the park. Set a group goal, such as a three-mile "walk for hunger" or some other worthy cause.

- **Mental checkpoints:** If your usual walk just seems too long, too daunting, break it up into smaller chunks in your mind. Start out by telling yourself that you'll just walk to the red bungalow several streets over with the pretty rose garden out front, the quarter point of your walk. You could turn around and head home, but instead try for another checkpoint, the intersection with the flashing yellow traffic light that marks the halfway point. Now that you've made it this far, it's just as far to turn around and head home as it is to keep going, so why not push onward, past the neighborhood eyesore that marks the three-quarter point and all the way home? Just as it helps

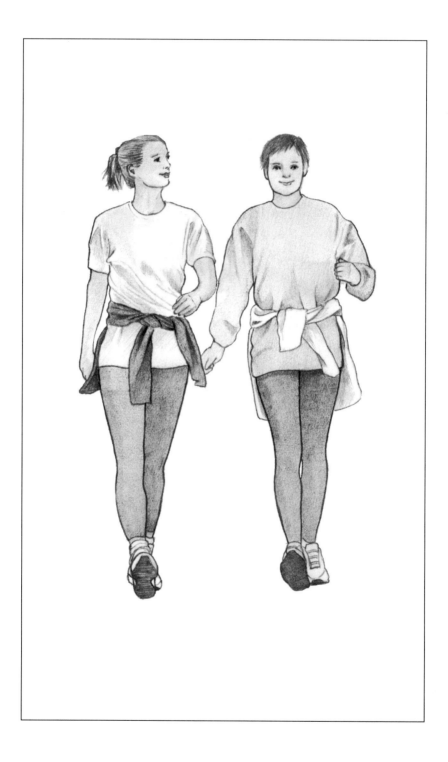

to break a larger goal into smaller, more achievable portions, thinking of your walk or exercise routine in smaller, more manageable sections may help you get out the door and get started on days when you'd rather sit at home.

- **Cognitive restructuring:** Try replacing negative thoughts you might have toward exercise with positive thoughts of your ability to carry through with your exercise plan. Rather than thinking, "I hate to walk, I don't want to do this," tell yourself, "I've done this dozens of times before, and I remember how good it made me feel afterward. I can do this today." In Chapter 1, we asked you to take the "Lifestyle Inventory." To remind yourself of how good your healthy lifestyle makes you feel, retake it whenever you have trouble getting started, and compare your answers to those from Chapter 1.

Do these tools work? Joan, the 38-year-old attorney we met in Chapter 3, routinely uses visualization/mental imagery and cognitive restructuring to get herself going. "I've had relapses, but I won't let them derail me for long periods any more. Usually, I feel so good at the end of a workout—and I know that now—so that's the motivation. If I'm going through a really bad day I can stop for a minute and imagine how good I'll feel later when I am exercising, and I'll feel better. People starting out don't know that, so it's hard for them to picture the payoff."

In time, the positive feelings that result from your workouts will become so dominant they will motivate you to get going when it's a challenge to do so. For Joan, exercise itself has become the reward.

Points to Remember

- Take rewards seriously—they help you to form positive associations with exercise. Don't neglect them.
- Relapses in exercise do occur. When they do, take them in stride and focus on getting started once again.

"It's all to do with the training: you can do a lot if you're
properly trained."

Elizabeth II (1926–), Queen of England

8

Three Strength-Training Workouts

The strength-training exercises we will present in this chapter draw on three programs developed by Fatima Valeras, a Boston-based fitness instructor and personal trainer. The differences among the programs are described below:

- **15-Minute Strength Essentials:** for women who have done no strength training at all and would like to build their muscles for functional fitness
- **20-Minute Total Body Basics:** for women who want to build their strength further
- **20-Minute Quick Intervals:** for women who cannot walk outside on a particular day or who have limited time for exercise. It includes both strength training and aerobic exercise in one program (the "intervals" refer to the aerobic exercises)

The boxes that accompany each program include instructions for beginning, intermediate, and advanced readers, plus some helpful guidelines and tips for proper technique and form.

BOX 38

15-Minute Strength Essentials: Guidelines and Tips

- **Purpose and requirements**: Emphasizes functionality and requires little or no equipment.
- **Beginner**: Perform 8–10 repetitions, one set per exercise.
- **Intermediate:** Perform 10–12 repetitions, two sets per exercise.
- **Advanced:** Perform 12–15 repetitions, two sets per exercise.
- **Posture:** For every exercise, hold your stomach muscles tight to help support the trunk. Breathe naturally. For standing exercises, keep your head up and eyes forward. For exercises on your back, look up at the ceiling; for those on your stomach, look down at the floor.
- **Execution:** Each exercise repetition should take approximately 7 seconds to complete. Each stretch should be held for 20–30 seconds. Counting out loud helps.
- **Note**: Be sure to stretch the body part indicated after you complete this program of exercises. Use the stretching exercises at the end of this chapter.

BOX 39

15-Minute Strength Essentials: Purpose of Each Exercise

Exercise	Target	Stretch/Tone
Wall squat	Lower body	Front and back of thighs
Lunge	Hips, buttocks	Front, back, and inner thighs, calves
Bent-knee sit-up, hyperextension	Lower back, abdominals	Abs, lower back
Modified push-up, dip	Shoulders, arms	Upper body, shoulders, chest, upper back

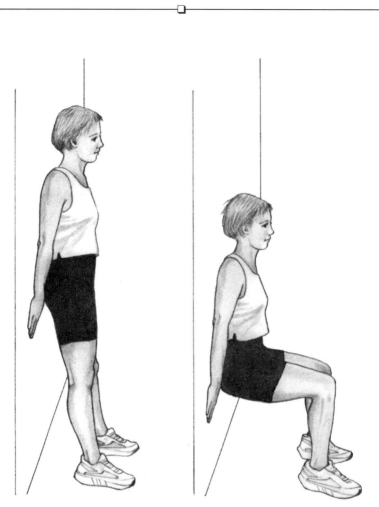

- **Wall squat:** With your feet a shoulder's width apart and your knees slightly bent, stand thigh-distance from a wall. Holding your shoulder blades together, press the length of your back against the wall. Lower your thighs until they are parallel, or nearly parallel, to the floor. Keep your hips at knee level or higher. Hold for four counts and press up from the heels to start position. Option: Squat with arms extended in front for balance.

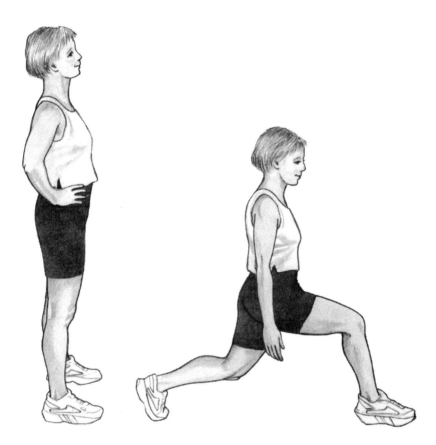

▪ **Lunge:** Stand with your legs a shoulder's width apart, with your shoulders back and down (instead of hunched) and your hands on your hips. Step forward with your right leg and plant one heel directly under your knee. While in place, roll your back foot on its ball. Balancing in this 90° position, lower your front thigh until it is parallel, or nearly parallel, to the floor. Keep your hip at knee level, and not lower. Press up from the right heel to start position. Repeat with other side. Option: Extend your arms to the sides, or in front, for balance.

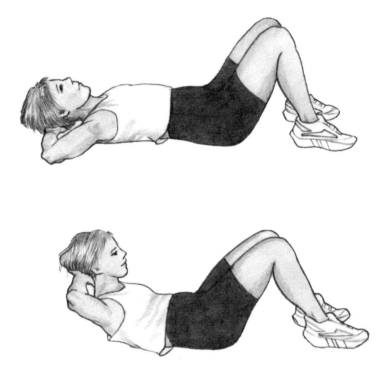

- **Bent-knee sit-up:** Lie on your back, and bend your knees to a point where your heels rest about a foot from your buttocks. Place your fingertips behind your head, with your chin off your chest. Curl your upper body an inch off the floor, squeezing your abdominal muscles. Exhale as you lift your shoulders and hold this "crunch" for two counts. Inhale as you release the squeeze halfway to the floor. Option: Instead of placing your fingertips behind your head, extend your arms over your thighs and curl your upper body until your fingertips reach your knees.

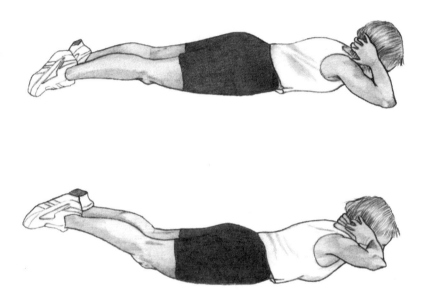

- **Hyperextension:** Lie face down with the front of your feet flat on the floor. Place your fingers behind your ears and lift your head and chest an inch off the floor. Hold the pull for two counts, then release to start position. If this exercise is too difficult, use the hyperextension described on page 143.

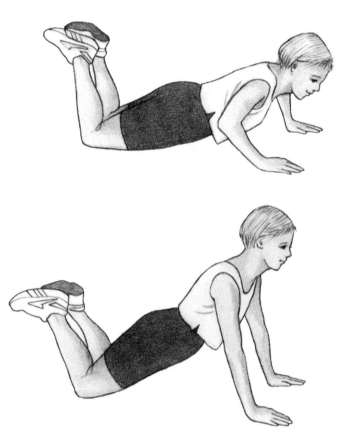

• **Modified push-up:** On your knees, lie face down and place your hands a shoulder's width apart, palms flat next to your chest. Bring your trunk/body up in one unit by pressing your arms into a straight position, hands under your shoulders. Lower it by bending the arms and bringing the chest close to, but not down on, the floor. Repeat without touching the floor with your chest. Option: Do these push-ups against a wall, feet together and toes about a foot from the wall.

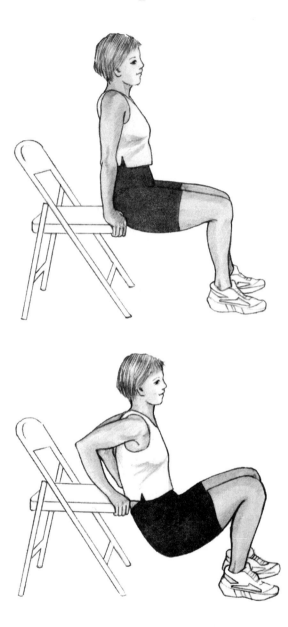

• **Dip:** Sit at the end of a chair, holding onto the front of it with both hands. Position your feet in front, a shoulder's width apart. Keeping your back close to the edge of the chair, lower your torso until your upper arms are parallel to the floor. Push up slowly, using your arms (and not your legs) and return to the starting position.

BOX 40

20-Minute Total Body Basics: Guidelines and Tips

- **Purpose and requirements:** Emphasizes strength and requires a weighted bar or a pair of dumbbells and a chair.
- **Beginner:** Perform 8–10 repetitions, one set per exercise.
- **Intermediate:** Perform 10–12 repetitions, two sets per exercise.
- **Advanced:** Using weights perform 12–15 repetitions, two sets per exercise.
- **Posture:** For every exercise, hold the stomach muscles tight to help support the trunk, and breathe naturally. For standing exercises, keep the head up and the eyes forward. For exercises that are to be done on your back, look up at the ceiling; for those on your stomach, look down at the floor.
- **Execution:** Each exercise repetition should take approximately 7 seconds to complete. Each stretch should be held for 20–30 seconds. Counting out loud helps.
- **Note:** Be sure to stretch the body part indicated after you complete this program of exercises. Use the stretching exercises at the end of this chapter.

BOX 41

20-Minute Total Body Basics: Purpose of Each Exercise

Exercise	Target	Stretch/Tone
Dumbbell squat, step-up, calf raise	Legs	Front and back of thighs, calves
Bent-over row, back fly	Back	Shoulders, upper back
Dumbbell curl, tricep extension	Arms	Upper body
Chest press, chest fly	Chest	Upper body, chest, shoulders
Shoulder press, upright row	Shoulder	Shoulders, arms
Crunch, hyperextension	Abdominals, lower back	Abs, lower back

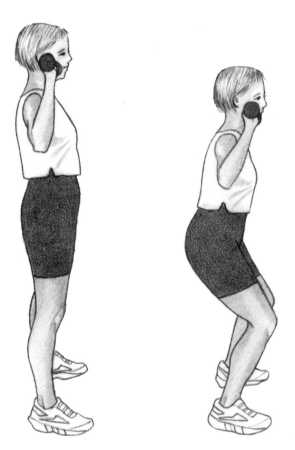

- **Dumbbell squat:** Stand with your feet slightly wider than a shoulder's width apart, knees slightly bent. With your back straight, shoulders back and down (rather than hunched), hold dumbbells one of two ways—either at your sides with arms extended or behind your neck and shoulders with the dumbbells parallel to the floor. Lower your thighs until they are parallel, or nearly parallel, to the floor (as if you were sitting in a chair). Keep your knees at hip level or above, but not lower. Hold for a count of three, making sure that your knees track directly over your shoelaces. To finish, press up from your heels to return to the start position.

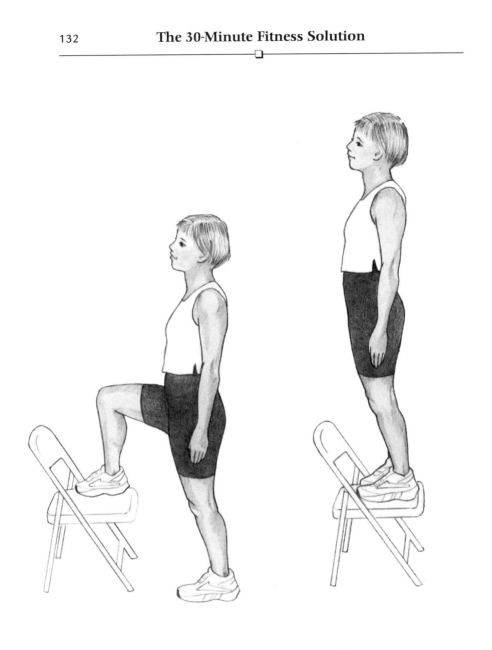

- **Step-up:** With your arms extended by your sides, step onto an adjustable step or bench with a heel-to-toe motion, with one foot following the other. Stand straight when stepping up, then reverse the procedure, rocking the ball of your foot to your heel as you step back down to the start position. Alternate the leg that starts the process.

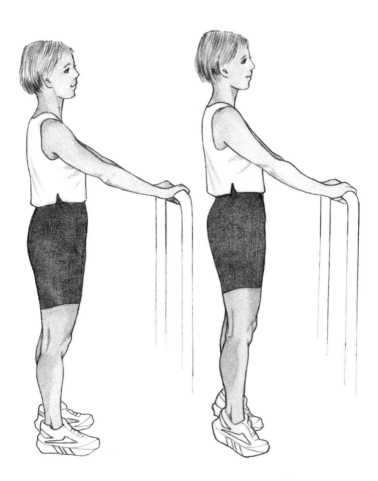

• **Calf raise:** Using a bar or a chair back for support, stand with your feet together and squeeze the lower leg muscles by raising yourself onto your toes. Roll back to the heels and repeat.

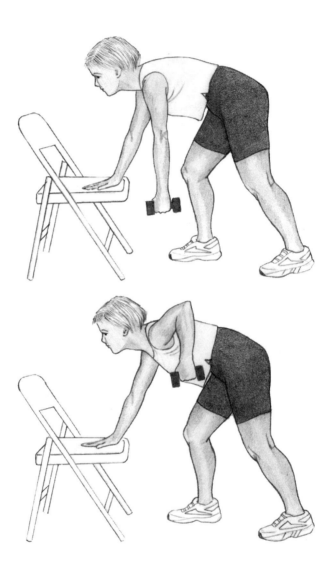

- **Bent-over row:** With your feet slightly wider than a shoulder's width apart, bend your knees and hinge forward from the hip so your torso becomes parallel with the floor. Hold dumbbells about a shoulder's width apart, with arms extended under the shoulders. Bring the elbows back toward the ceiling, keeping the back flat and the elbows close to the ribcage. Hold for a count of three and return the bar to the start position.

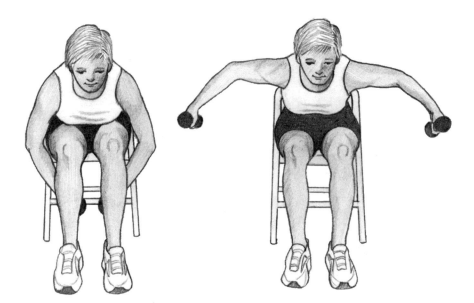

- **Back fly:** Seated at the end of a step or bench, rest the chest on the thighs and place the dumbbells underneath the thighs. With the palms facing in, raise the dumbbells behind you so that your elbows point to the ceiling and your arms extend to the sides. Squeeze the middle back muscle for a count of three, then return to the start position.

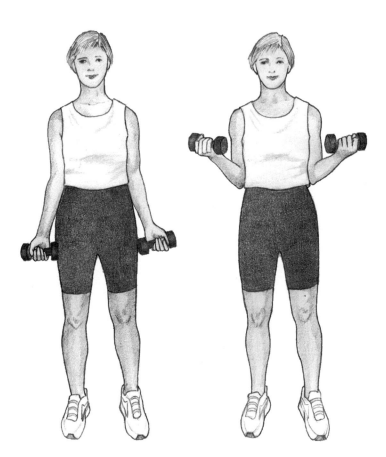

- **Dumbbell curl:** Stand with your feet a shoulder's width apart, knees slightly bent, shoulders back and down, with the dumbbells palm side up. Keeping your upper arms stationary, bend your elbows and bring the dumbbells to shoulder level without swinging the back. Pause for one count and return the dumbbells to the start position.

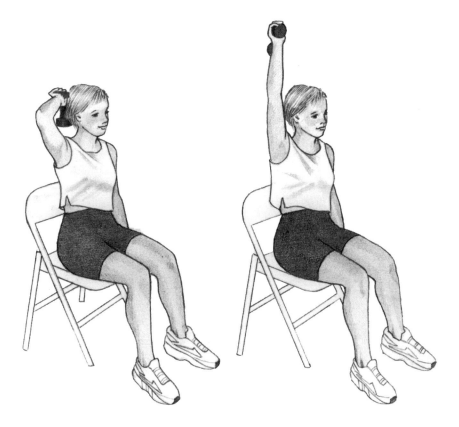

- **Tricep extension:** Hold a dumbbell by its end in one hand. Raise the weight above your head so your palms face up and the weight is perpendicular to the floor. Keeping your elbow close to your head, bend your forearm back to 90° and then extend the arm back to the start position. Repeat with the other arm.

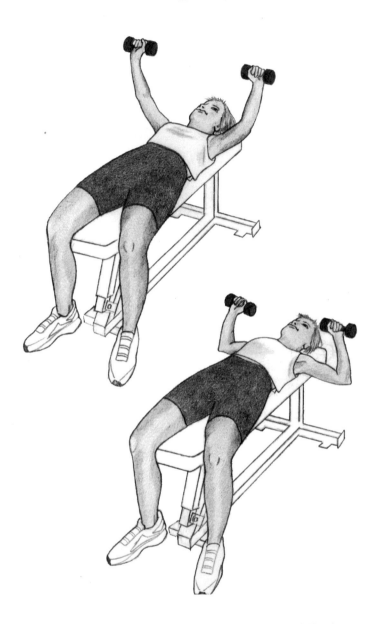

- **Chest press:** Grab the dumbbells, palms down, and lie down on a bench with your back and hips pressed firmly to the bench. Extend your arms straight above your shoulders, palms facing your feet, then lower the weight by bending your elbows so your upper arms are parallel to the floor, about 90°. Press the weight back up to the starting position.

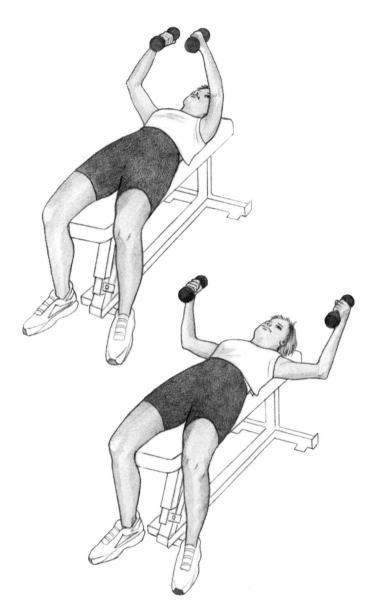

• **Chest fly:** With a dumbbell in each hand, lie on a bench and press your hips and back into the bench with your palms fairly close together. Extend your arms, palms facing one another, and lower your arms to your sides so your elbows point to the floor. Extend far back enough to feel a stretch in the chest, then bring the weights back to the palms-together position.

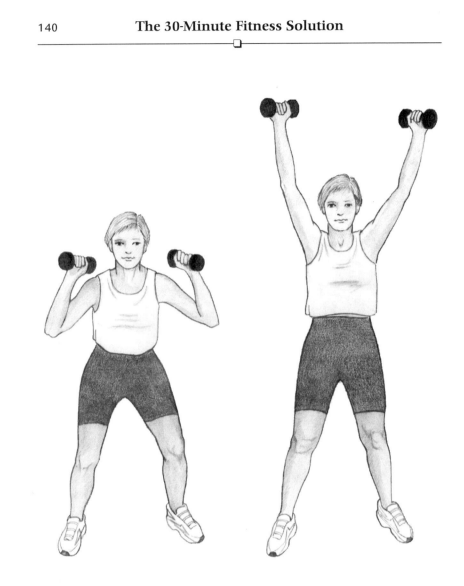

- **Shoulder press:** With the knees bent, feet a shoulder's width apart, and back straight, place the dumbbells on your shoulders, palms facing away. Press the weight above your head by extending your arms but not locking your elbows. Return the weight to shoulder level and repeat.

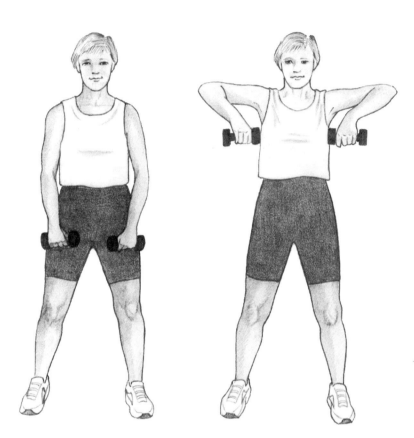

• **Upright row:** Standing with your feet a shoulder's width apart, knees bent, back straight, shoulders down and back, hold a dumbbell in each hand, palms side down, in front of your thighs. With your arms extended and the weight close to your body, bring your elbows up and out to the side. The weight should come up no higher than chest level.

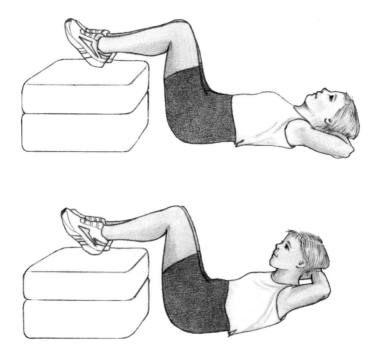

- **Crunch:** Lie on your back with your feet on top of a step or bench. Your legs should form a 90° angle at the hips. Place your fingertips behind your head and with your chin off your chest, lift your shoulders off the floor about an inch or so to contract the abdominal muscles. Keep your hips steady and your lower back on the floor. Hold at the peak for two counts then return to the start position.

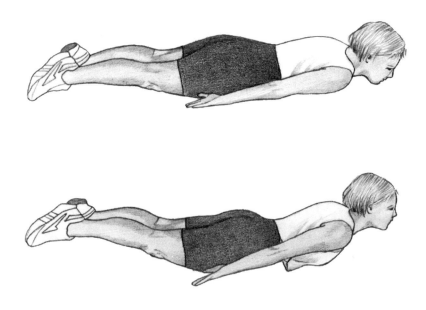

- **Hyperextension:** Lie face down with the front of your feet flat on the floor. Extend your arms at your sides and lift your chest and head an inch or two off the floor.

BOX 42

20-Minute Quick Intervals: Guidelines and Tips

- **Purpose and equipment:** Emphasizes functional fitness and strength and requires little or no equipment.
- **Beginner, intermediate, and advanced:** Perform one set of 20 repetitions per strength exercise.
- **Posture:** For every exercise, hold your stomach muscles tight to help support your trunk. Breathe naturally. For standing exercises, keep your head up and your eyes forward. For exercises on your back, imagine that you are pulling your navel through the floor; for those on your stomach, look down at the floor.
- **Execution:** Each exercise should take approximately two minutes to complete. Move from strength training to aerobic exercise with little or no break in between.
- **Note:** Be sure to stretch after each session, using the stretching exercises at the end of this chapter.

BOX 43

20-Minute Quick Intervals: Purpose of Each Exercise

Exercise	Target	Stretch/Tone
One minute of aerobic exercise (jump rope, cycle, walk, and so on)	Warm-up	Activity-specific
Military press	Strength	Front and back of thighs, buttocks, shoulders, arms
Three minutes (running in place, rope-skipping, or cycling)	Cardiovascular	Activity-specific
Lunge-curl	Strength	Front and back of thighs, arms, upper body
Three minutes (running in place, rope-skipping, or cycling)	Cardiovascular	Activity-specific
Modified push-up	Strength	Upper body, shoulders, chest
Three minutes (running in place, rope-skipping, or cycling)	Cardiovascular	Activity-specific
Oblique crunch	Strength	Abdominal area, lower back
Two minutes	Cool down	Activity-specific

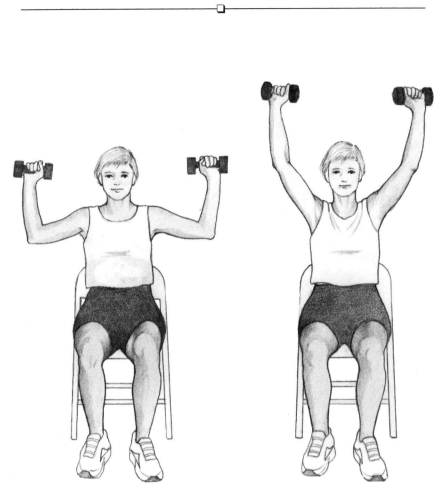

• **Military press:** Sit in a chair, with your feet a shoulder's width apart and your back straight and firm against the chair. Hold the dumbbells level with your ears, with your palms facing forward. Lift the dumbbells toward the ceiling, keeping a slight bend in your elbows. Slowly lower the weight to the starting position.

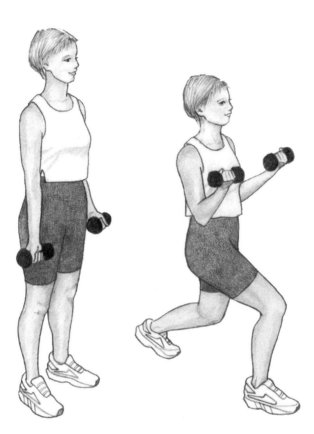

- **Lunge curl:** Stand with your feet a shoulder's width apart, with your shoulders back and down, instead of hunched. With your arms extended by your sides, hold two dumbbells in your hands, palms facing away. Begin the lunge by stepping forward with your right leg, and planting your heal directly under your right knee. Still in place, your left foot should roll on the ball to form a 90° position with your knees. As your right thigh lowers to become parallel or nearly parallel to the floor, bend your elbows and lift the weight upward with a curling motion from your thighs to your shoulders. Do not exceed hip to knee level or touch the back knee to the floor. Press up from the right heel to return to the starting position, and lower your arms to hip level. Alternate legs and repeat.

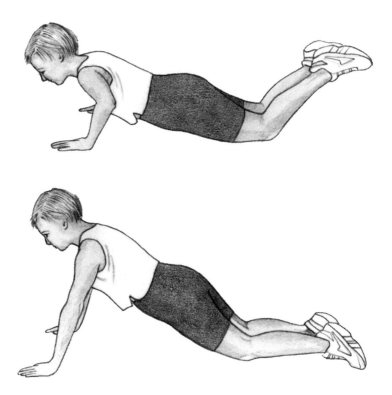

- **Modified push-up:** Get down on the floor on all fours, with your arms shoulder-width apart and your palms flat next to your chest. Lower and raise your trunk in one unit, making sure that you come close to the floor, but do not rest on it.

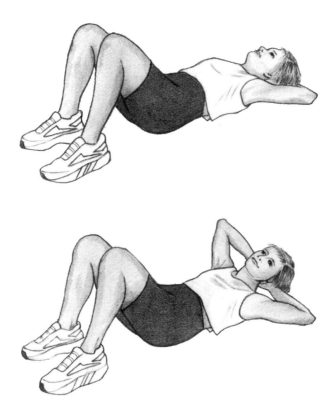

- **Oblique crunch:** Lie on your back with your legs up, knees bent, making sure that your legs form a 90° angle at your hips. Place your fingertips behind your ears, making sure that your chin is off of your chest. Lift one shoulder about one inch off the floor toward the opposite knee (you should feel your abdominal muscles contract). As you do this, make sure you keep your hips steady and your lower back on the floor. Hold this position for two counts and then return to start. Alternate the shoulder-knee combination.

Stretch for a Healthy Body

While it is important to rest two days between strength-training sessions, stretching, on the other hand, can—and should—be done every day to help you stay limber and avoid injury.

Stretching is important for anyone, from the 20-year-old to the 70-year-old, emphasizes strength-training expert Wayne Westcott. "Unfortunately, most people don't start stretching until they have an injury." Why wait for an injury to start stretching? Wouldn't it be better to make stretching and flexibility exercises a part of your day right now, so you can retain your full range of motion and balance for all of your life?

Try doing the simple stretching exercises in this chapter twice a day. It helps if you initially link them with some other activity you do each day, like brushing your teeth or changing from your work clothes. You'll quickly note that they take very little time to complete—5 to 10 minutes for each session. But don't rush. Be sure to do them slowly—hold each position for 20 to 30 seconds—without bouncing, so you can feel the muscle gently and easily give way to the stretch.

Here are some stretching exercise for home or office. They are adapted from a program developed by Michael Wood, CSCS, Director of the Sports Performance Group in Cambridge, Massachusetts.

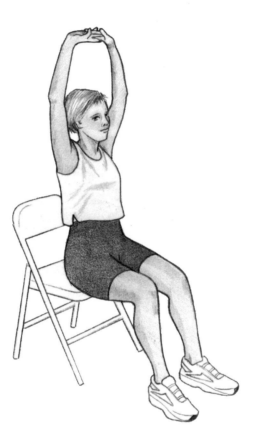

- **Reach for the stars:** For the shoulders and upper back. Sit up straight on the front edge of your chair. Interlock your fingers and extend your arms upward, pressing your palms toward the ceiling, holding for a minimum of 15 seconds. Keep your shoulders behind your ears and your eyes straight.

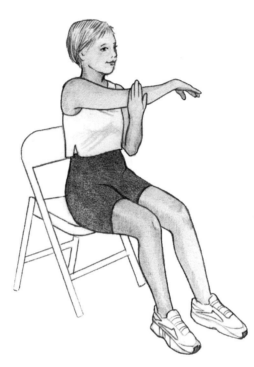

- **Arm pull:** For the shoulders. Once again, sit up straight on the edge of a chair. Bring your left arm across your chest. With your right hand, gently pull your left elbow toward your chin and hold for 15 seconds. Switch arms and repeat.

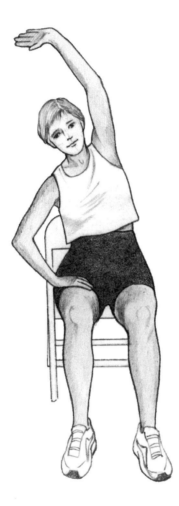

▪ **Side stretch:** For the trunk, obliques, and shoulders. Sitting erect in your chair, reach for the ceiling with your right hand. You should feel a stretch along the rib cage as well as in the trunk and waist areas. Now, slowly flex your trunk from the left side.

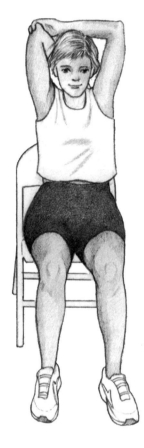

- **Elbow point:** For the arms, chest, and shoulders. Once again, as you are sitting, point your left elbow toward the ceiling, then bring your fingers toward your right shoulder blade. Bring your right hand up to your left elbow and gently push the elbow back, and hold for 15–30 seconds. Switch arms and repeat.

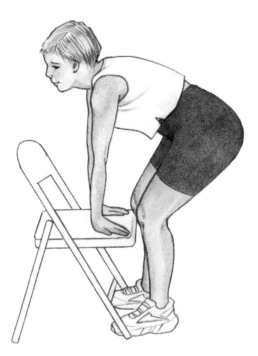

• **Wrist stretch:** For the wrist flexors. While standing, place both hands palms-down on a flat surface with your fingers pointing toward your body. Keep your palms on a flat surface and your arms straight, then try to move your body back slightly. You will feel a strong stretch up the forearm and wrist areas.

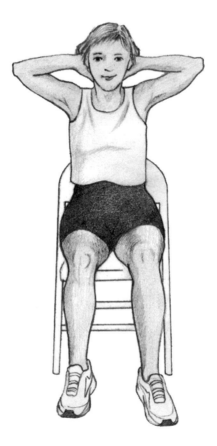

- **Chest stretch:** For the chest and shoulders. Back to your chair, sit erectly, with your feet on the floor. Interlock you hands behind your head. Slowly pull your elbows back, keeping your hands interlocked throughout the stretch.

Points to Remember

▪ These efficient strength-training programs are designed to help you fit strength training into your busy day. Start with the 15-Minute Strength-Training Essentials, then graduate to 20-Minute Total Body Basics.

▪ Use the 20-Minute Quick Intervals on days when you can't get outside to exercise or have limited time to fit it in.

▪ And try to stretch every day! It will help keep you limber and reduce tension.

9

Home Equipment and Health Clubs

Let's be practical: you'll have days when you just can't go outside and walk for 30 minutes—for any number of reasons. You may oversleep in the morning, get home too late at night, or find that the pressing needs of a child, parent, spouse, or friend take precedence over exercising. Your area may be socked with a rain storm, a heat wave, or a blizzard. In other words, "life" gets in the way of your exercise routine.

To remedy that situation, you might want to consider purchasing a piece of home exercise equipment to fall back on. That way, you can exercise completely at your own convenience—at any time of the day or night, regardless of last-minute changes in your schedule or the weather.

Lots of people go the home-exercise route. According to a recent survey, odds are that either you or one of your immediate neighbors owns an exercise machine. These machines are big business, with sales in the neighborhood of $5 billion a year. The rub is that many people never get around to using what they buy—at least not on a regular basis. Almost a third of people who buy exercise machines don't use them.

How can you make sure you aren't buying yourself an expensive coat rack? Purchasing the right piece of equipment is the first important step. To buy well, you need to know what kinds of exercises you like—and don't like—to do; how much space you have available; and

158

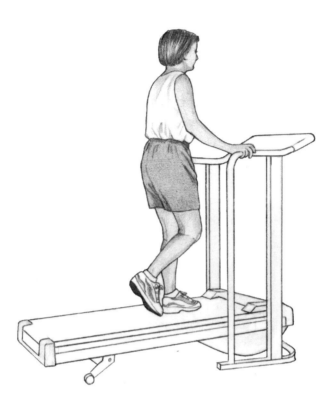

what kind of options you want. In other words, plan carefully before buying. One of the best investments you can make is trying out a variety of different machines at a local health club.

The Fitness Products Council, a trade organization that represents manufacturers and distributors of exercise machines and other fitness products, suggests the following guidelines to consider before buying an exercise machine:

- **Commit to your goals:** Know what you want to accomplish and exactly how an exercise machine will help you fulfill those goals.
- **Know what you like:** Instead of buying a machine in hope that its presence in your home will get you started exercising, try out different machines to find out which ones suit your style (see Box 44). You can do so with a short-term membership at a health club or by using a friend's equipment. You can also don your workout clothes and test out the equipment at a store.

BOX 44

Choosing a Home Exercise Machine

Type	Advantages	Disadvantages	What to Look For	Cost
Treadmill	Good approximation of outdoor walking or running; may be easier on the joints than running on hard pavement; provides weight-bearing workout; some fold for easy storage	May be more expensive and more prone to breaking down than other kinds of machines	Make sure the belt of the treadmill is long enough and wide enough for your stride; front and side rails; an emergency stop device	Under $400 to $2,500+; cheaper models may not be good for runners or for heavy people
Exercise bicycle	Easy to use without any training; need minimal balance and coordination; you can read or watch TV while riding; durable	Most models don't work the upper body; not a weight-bearing form of exercise, so it won't strengthen bones; can get uncomfortable during long workouts	Get an adjustable, comfortable seat; if you have high blood pressure, test a recumbent bike; toe clips are worth getting for the pedals	$200 to $2,000
Ski machine	Generally easy on the knees; works both the upper and lower body; good ones really simulate cross-country skiing	Dependent motion machines (pushing one ski forward makes the other move backward) can be awkward, while independent motion machines can take time to master	Machines with ropes can give you a more natural workout than machines with immovable handgrips	$100 to $700+

BOX 44 (cont.)

Rowing machine	Offers as close to a full-body workout as a machine can provide	Unfamiliar motion; can be hard on the knees or back	Pulley models offer a more realistic rowing experience than piston models	$200 to $1,000
Elliptical exerciser	Offers as close to a no-impact workout as a machine can provide; can mimic walking or cross-country skiing; easier on the joints than a treadmill	May take some time to get used to; workout may be too hard for beginners, not hard enough for well-conditioned exercisers	Nonslip pedals with curved ridges to hold your feet in place; comfortable handlebars	$500 to $4,000+
Stairstepper	A low-impact workout that lets you read or watch TV while working out	Some people find it to be too strenuous at first; can be hard on the knees	Machines with independent foot action give a more realistic feel; handrails and large stair platforms are important safety features	$200 to $1,500+

- **Measure your space:** You'll be more likely to exercise if you put your machine in a pleasant, in-the-way spot. Keep in mind that some machines can take up a lot of space. At the store, you'll want to ask about the machine's "footprint," or the amount of room it takes up on the floor.
- **Remember, you get what you pay for:** When testing machines, try out the top-of-the-line model and work your way down. The most expensive one will show you what sorts of bells and whistles you don't need, while giving you a good idea of how a high-quality machine should feel.
- **Don't expect one machine to do everything:** A single exercise machine probably can't give you aerobic conditioning, weight-resistance training, and stretching. That means you'll either need to buy several machines or supplement the one machine with other kinds of free exercises.
- **Listen to the machine:** Really. You want to be able to hear yourself think, or hear something else—like a radio, the television, or a conversation.
- **Buy for the future:** Make sure your machine comes with a written warranty, and that the manufacturer has a customer service telephone number for your questions. Ask about the seller's policies regarding installation, maintenance, and service.

Copies of the Fitness Products Council's pamphlet, "How to Buy Exercise Equipment for the Home" is available on the Internet at http://www.sportlink.com/research/1998_research/fitness/98_home_gym_guide.html or by sending an email request to the Council at sdsgma@aol.com.

Getting Started with Home Exercise Equipment

Okay. You have your new equipment set up at home, in a comfortable spot. Perhaps in front of the television, or near your stereo, so you can entertain yourself a bit as you exercise. How much should you exercise today, your first day? How do you progress safely in the weeks ahead, so you'll be challenged, but you won't end up sore and discouraged, ready to quit?

To answer that, you need a *program to follow*. Fortunately, a growing number of equipment manufacturers are putting exercise programs on the Internet to get you started using your new piece of equipment. To find such a program, check the product literature for the manufacturer's Web site. Or ask the sales person in the store. You may also find it by going to www.Yahoo.com and searching by typing in the company's name. If the company does have a Web site, it should show up as one of the matching entries.

Keep in mind that there are also a growing number of independent fitness Web sites that provide personal programs and online coaching for you. To find a listing of such sites, go to www.Yahoo.com again and click on the health and fitness link. You'll find a number of useful sites there, including http://www.About.com, and http://www.Fitnessfind.com, both of which provide numerous additional links. While some Web sites listed will provide actual programs, others are mostly informational. They'll tell you everything you ever wanted to know about the home fitness activity you're pursuing. Many also have chat rooms so you can share information and tips with other home exercisers.

Since lots of people aren't quite as computer-savvy as they would like to be, we asked Michael Wood to create exercise programs for four of the most popular home-exercise machines—treadmill, exercise bicycle, rowing machine, and stair-stepper (Box 45). These programs are designed especially for beginners, to help you progress slowly and steadily, so you can build up the frequency, intensity, and duration you spend exercising without experiencing discomfort.

How to Choose a Health Club

Between 1987 and 1995, the number of health club members in the United States nearly doubled, reports the International Health, Racquet and Sportsclub Association (IHRSA), the largest fitness trade association worldwide, with more than 3,200 member clubs in the United States and 2,000 abroad. Once thought to be the domain of the very young, health clubs now attract people of all ages. In fact, one in 10 members is age 65 or older

Why do people join health and sports clubs? The reasons people

BOX 45

8-Week Home Exercise Program

TREADMILL

Time = minutes   Speed = miles per hour   Heart rate: record at end of session

WEEK 1

Day 1	Time	Speed	Elevation	Heart rate	Day 2	Time	Speed	Elevation	Heart rate
Mon.	5	3	0%		Fri.	5	3.3	0%	
	3	3.3	3%			3	3.3	4%	
	3	3.3	4%			3	3.5	3%	
	4	3	0%			4	3.3	0%	
Total	15				Total	15			

WEEK 2

Day 1	Time	Speed	Elevation	Heart rate	Day 2	Time	Speed	Elevation	Heart rate
Mon.	5	3.3	0%		Fri.	5	3.3	0%	
	4	3.5	3%			4	3.5	4%	
	4	3.5	4%			4	3.5	4%	
	5	3.5	0%			5	3.3	0%	
Total	18				Total	18			

WEEK 3

Day 1	Time	Speed	Elevation	Heart rate	Day 2	Time	Speed	Elevation	Heart rate
Mon.	5	3	0%		Fri.	5	3.3	0%	
	5	3.3	3%			5	3.3	4%	
	5	3.3	4%			5	3.5	3%	
	5	3	0%			5	3.3	0%	
Total	20				Total	20			

BOX 45 (cont.)

WEEK 4

Days 1 & 3	Time	Speed	Elevation	Heart rate	Day 2	Time	Speed	Elevation	Heart rate
Mon.	5	3.3	0%		Wed.	3	3.3	0%	
Fri.	6	3.8	4%			3	3.8	4%	
	3	3.5	5%			3	3.5	4%	
	3	3.5	0%			3	3.5	0%	
Total	17				Total	12			

WEEK 5

Day 1	Time	Speed	Elevation	Heart rate	Day 2	Time	Speed	Elevation	Heart rate
Mon.	5	3.3	0%		Fri.	5	3.3	0%	
	6	3.5	4%			10	3.3	4%	
	6	3.8	5%			5	3.5	3%	
	6	3.3	0%			5	3.3	0%	
Total	23				Total	25			

WEEK 6

Days 1 & 3	Time	Speed	Elevation	Heart rate	Day 2	Time	Speed	Elevation	Heart rate
Mon.	5	3.3	0%		Wed.	5	3.3	0%	
Fri.	7	3.5	3%			8	3.5	4%	
	7	3.5	4%			8	3.5	4%	
	5	3.5	0%			5	3.3	0%	
Total	24				Total	26			

WEEK 7

Day 1	Time	Speed	Elevation	Heart rate	Day 2	Time	Speed	Elevation	Heart rate
Mon.	5	3	0%		Fri.	5	3.3	0%	
	10	3.3	3%			10	3.3	4%	
	7	3.3	4%			9	3.5	3%	
	5	3	0%			4	3.3	0%	
Total	27				Total	28			

BOX 45 (cont.)

WEEK 8

Days 1 & 3	Time	Speed	Elevation	Heart rate	Day 2	Time	Speed	Elevation	Heart rate
Mon.	5	3.5	0%		Wed.	5	3.5	0%	
Fri.	10	3.5	5%			10	3.8	6%	
	10	3.5	5%			10	4	4%	
	5	3.5	0%			5	3.5	0%	
Total	30				Total	30			

STAIR-STEPPER

Weeks 1–4: set on manual program   Weeks 5–8: set on hill program   Time = minutes
MET = metabolic energy table   Heart rate: record at end of session

WEEK 1

Day 1	Time	MET level	Heart rate	Day 2	Time	MET level	Heart rate
Mon.	3	2		Fri.	3	3	
	3	3			3	4	
	3	4			3	4	
	3	5			3	5	
Total	12			Total	12		

WEEK 2

Day 1	Time	MET level	Heart rate	Day 2	Time	MET level	Heart rate
Mon.	3	3		Fri.	3	4	
	4	4			4	5	
	4	5			4	6	
	4	6			4	5	
Total	15			Total	15		

WEEK 3

Day 1	Time	MET level	Heart rate	Day 2	Time	MET level	Heart rate
Mon.	7	2		Fri.	5	3	
	5	3			5	6	
	3	4			3	5	
	3	5			3	4	
Total	18			Total	16		

BOX 45 (cont.)

WEEK 4

Days 1 & 3	Time	MET level	Heart rate	Day 2	Time	MET level	Heart rate
Mon.	5	5		Wed.	5	4	
Fri.	5	5			5	6	
	5	5			5	7	
Total	15			Total	15		

WEEK 5

Day 1	Time	MET level	Heart rate	Day 2	Time	MET level	Heart rate
Mon.	20	6		Wed.	10	5	
					5	6	
					5	6	
					3	5	
Total	20			Total	23		

WEEK 6

Day 1	Time	MET level	Heart rate	Day 2	Time	MET level	Heart rate
Mon.	5	6		Fri.	OFF		
	5	6					
	5	6					
	5	6					
Total	20			Total			

WEEK 7

Day 1	Time	MET level	Heart rate	Day 2	Time	MET level	Heart rate
Mon.	25	7		Fri.	5	7	
					10	10	
					10	9	
					5	8	
Total	25			Total	30		

BOX 45 (cont.)

WEEK 8

Days 1 & 3	Time	MET level	Heart rate	Day 2	Time	MET level	Heart rate
Mon.	5	6		Wed.	5	7	
Fri.	10	8			5	10	
	5	8			10	8	
Total	20			Total	20		

EXERCISE BICYCLE

Time = minutes   Level = intensity of workout   RPM = revolutions per minute
Heart rate: record at end of session

WEEK 1

Day 1	Time	Level	RPM	Heart rate	Day 2	Time	Level	RPM	Heart rate
Mon.	5	2	60–65		Fri.	5	3	60–65	
	3	3	65			3	4	65	
	2	2	60			2	4	60	
Total	10				Total	10			

WEEK 2

Day 1	Time	Level	RPM	Heart rate	Day 2	Time	Level	RPM	Heart rate
Mon.	5	3	65		Fri.	5	4	65	
	4	4	65–70			6	4	70	
	3	3	65			3	4	70	
Total	12				Total	14			

WEEK 3

Day 1	Time	Level	RPM	Heart rate	Day 2	Time	Level	RPM	Heart rate
Mon.	5	4	70		Fri.	5	5	60–65	
	8	5	65			8	5	65	
	2	4	70			4	5	60	
Total	15				Total	17			

BOX 45 (cont.)

WEEK 4

Day 1	Time	Level	RPM	Heart rate	Day 2	Time	Level	RPM	Heart rate
Mon.	5	6	70		Fri.	5	6	70	
	8	5	70			8	6	75	
	5	6	70			7	6	70	
Total	18				Total	20			

WEEK 5

Days 1 & 3	Time	Level	RPM	Heart rate	Day 2	Time	Level	RPM	Heart rate
Mon.	5	7	70		Wed.	5	5	70	
Fri.	20	6	75			20	7	70	
						5	5	70	
Total	25				Total	30			

WEEK 6

Day 1	Time	Level	RPM	Heart rate	Day 2	Time	Level	RPM	Heart rate
Mon.	5	7	70		Fri.	5	6	75	
	25	8	75			25	8	75	
	5	6	70			5	7	70	
Total	35				Total	35			

WEEK 7

Days 1 & 3	Time	Level	RPM	Heart rate	Day 2	Time	Level	RPM	Heart rate
Mon.	5	7	70		Wed.	5	5	70	
Fri.	30	6	75			20	7	75	
	5	6	75			15	5	70	
Total	40				Total	40			

WEEK 8

Day 1	Time	Level	RPM	Heart rate	Day 2	Time	Level	RPM	Heart rate
Mon.	5	7	70		Fri.	5	6	75	
	35	8	80			35	8	80	
	5	6	70			5	7	70	
Total	45				Total	45			

BOX 45 (cont.)

ROWING MACHINE

Time = minutes　Distance = meters completed　SPM = strokes per minute
Damper = setting of flywheel (1-4 = skull; 6-10 = rowboat)　Heart rate (HR): record at end of session

WEEK 1

Day 1	Time	Dis-tance	SPM	Dam-per	HR	Day 2	Time	Dis-tance	SPM	Dam-per	HR
Mon.	5		24–26	1–5		Fri.	5		24–26	1–5	
Total	5					Total	5				

WEEK 2

Day 1	Time	Dis-tance	SPM	Dam-per	HR	Day 2	Time	Dis-tance	SPM	Dam-per	HR
Mon.	6		26	1–5		Fri.	7		26	2–5	
Total	6					Total	7				

WEEK 3

Day 1	Time	Dis-tance	SPM	Dam-per	HR	Day 2	Time	Dis-tance	SPM	Dam-per	HR
Mon.	4		25	3		Fri.	4		26	3	
	4		26				4		26	3	
Total	8			3		Total	8				

WEEK 4

Day 1	Time	Dis-tance	SPM	Dam-per	HR	Day 2	Time	Dis-tance	SPM	Dam-per	HR
Mon.	4		26	3		Fri.	6		26	3	
	6		25	4			6		27	4	
Total	10					Total	12				

WEEK 5

Days 1 & 3	Time	Dis-tance	SPM	Dam-per	HR	Day 2	Time	Dis-tance	SPM	Dam-per	HR
Mon.		500 m	26	5		Wed.		600 m	26	5	
Fri.		500 m	26	5		Inter-vals		600 m	27	5	
Total		1000 m				Total		1200 m			

BOX 45 (cont.)

WEEK 6

Days 1 & 3	Time	Dis-tance	SPM	Dam-per	HR	Day 2	Time	Dis-tance	SPM	Dam-per	HR
Mon.		750 m	27	6		Wed.		500 m	27	5	
Fri.		600 m	27	6		Inter-vals		500 m	26	5	
								500 m	25	4	
Total		1350 m				Total		1500 m			

WEEK 7

Days 1 & 3	Time	Dis-tance	SPM	Dam-per	HR	Day 2	Time	Dis-tance	SPM	Dam-per	HR
Mon.		750 m	27	1–5		Wed.		800 m	25+	5	
Fri.		750 m	27	1–5		Inter-vals		850 m	25+	5	
Total		1500 m						1650 m			

WEEK 8

Day 1	Time	Dis-tance	SPM	Dam-per	HR	Day 2	Time	Dis-tance	SPM	Dam-per	HR
Mon.		500 m	26	6		Fri.		2000 m	26+	5	
Inter-vals		500 m	26	6							
		500 m	26	6							
Total		1500 m				Total		2000 m			

give range from social support to safety to physical education (see Box 46).

How do you find a club that's right for you? IHRSA studies show that you will be more likely to use a club if it is convenient to your home or place of business. The best club referrals often come from family, friends, physicians, and co-workers. You can locate an IHRSA club by calling 1–800–766–1278, toll free (U.S. and Canada only) or by visiting www.healthclubs.com. At this site you can search

BOX 46

Why People Join Health and Sports Clubs

- To exercise regularly in a motivating and energizing environment
- To get the support they need to stay with an exercise program
- To learn a new sport—or continue playing a favorite sport—such as tennis, racquetball, basketball, or swimming
- To work out on a variety of user-friendly cardiovascular and resistance equipment
- To receive one-on-one guidance and support from qualified fitness professionals
- To exercise in a safe environment where CPR, emergency response, and other safeguards are available
- To have a place to exercise when it is too hot, too cold, or weather conditions are hazardous
- To improve their health and well-being through programs such as stress management, weight management, and smoking cessation
- To maintain strength, mobility and functionality throughout life
- To improve physical mobility through physical therapy and programs designed for people with special challenges, such as arthritis or osteoporosis
- To encourage their children to develop the life-long practice of exercising regularly
- To take advantage of child care programs, summer camps, and special activities geared towards children
- To meet old friends and make new friends through organized, off-site club activities such as hiking and skiing trips
- To take advantage of social activities such as dances, parties and picnics
- To make new friends

Source: Adapted from International Health, Racquet & Sportsclub Association

U.S., Canadian, and international health clubs and spas by equipment and programs offered.

The Web site http://www.healthclubs.com also features a powerful proximity and mapping service, so if you are trying to find a club in your home town, or in a strange city, you'll have a map to guide you. If you are traveling, the IHRSA Passport Program offers guest privileges at member clubs around the world.

Before signing up at a health club, make an appointment to tour the facilities. Visit the club during the hours that you are most likely to use it, and take the time to decide if you feel comfortable in the facility. While on the tour, ask your guide to let you spend some time alone talking to current members. As you tour the club and talk with people, use the checklist in Box 47 to help you determine if the club will be able to meet your fitness, social, and safety needs.

What You Should Know before Signing a Membership Agreement

If you choose to become a member of a club, you can expect to sign an agreement, indicating the length and terms of membership, as well as payment procedures and club policies. Be sure to:

- Examine the agreement carefully. Make sure all verbal agreements are spelled out in writing.
- Understand the length of term. Are you agreeing to a multi-year membership, an annual membership, or a month-to-month membership? Do not agree to sign up for a lifetime membership; they are illegal in most states.
- Know the cancellation policy. Thirty-seven states specifically regulate the maximum length of these contracts and cancellation provisions. To find out the applicable laws in your state, call your state consumer protection agency or attorney general's office.
- Be aware that it is standard policy to offer a "cooling off" period. This period is usually the three days after signing up for a membership, during which you may cancel the agreement without penalty. You may also want to check to see what other cancellation provisions are in the contract, provided by law, so you know the policy

BOX 47

Checklist for Evaluating a Health Club

- Are staff members friendly and helpful?
- Is the club clean and well maintained?
- Do fitness staff members have appropriate educational back-grounds or certification from nationally recognized certifying agencies?
- Are new members provided with a club orientation and instruction on how to use the equipment?
- Does the club have the cardiovascular resistance equipment you want and need to achieve your fitness goals?
- Does the club offer a sufficient number and variety of programs for you to achieve your fitness goals (aerobic, racquet sports, basketball, and so on)?
- Does the club offer instruction in a sport or activity that you might want to learn (tennis, squash, swimming, and so on)?
- Does the club offer a sufficient number and variety of programs for you to achieve other goals (stress management, weight management, smoking cessation, social activities)?
- Are there long lines at the equipment, or crowded aerobics classes, at the time that you would be using the club?
- Is childcare available if you need it?
- Is there adequate parking available if you need it?

Source: Adapted from International Health, Racquet & Sportsclub Association

in case you become disabled, change jobs, or change your residence.

- Ask if the club will "own" your contract, or if they will sell it to a third party. In the latter case, the club may have less incentive to provide good service and encouragement to stay with your exercise program. Also, it can be difficult to cancel a contract when a third party takes over.

- Check with the Better Business Bureau to see if complaints have been filed against the club.

Points to Remember

- Home exercise equipment can come in handy on days when you can't walk or do other exercise outside.
- To avoid purchasing what later amounts to an expensive coat rack, you'll need to shop wisely.
- Before buying, try out equipment first—either at a store, at a friend's house, or through a short-term membership at a health club.
- Use the programs in this chapter to get started with your equipment.
- A health club can also provide an alternative exercise environment.
- You'll want to shop wisely there, too, looking for a club that is convenient, well-managed, and staffed with certified trainers.

10

Eating Your Way to Good Health

If "we are what we eat," then America is white bread, beef, whole milk, cakes/cookies/donuts, and soft drinks. Those are the top five sources of calories in our diet, a snapshot compiled by researchers at the National Cancer Institute who surveyed almost 4,000 adults about their eating habits. The next five aren't much better: chicken, cheese, salad dressings/mayonnaise/margarine, and sugars/syrups/jams. The only vegetable to make the top 15 is the lowly potato, which makes an appearance at number 12.

It's not that we don't know what makes a healthy diet. That ageless exhortation from our parents, "Will you *please* eat your vegetables!" (the one we hear ourselves repeating with our own children), still stands as one of the centerpieces of good nutrition. The U.S. government and a variety of health organizations spend millions of dollars a year conveying the gospel of good nutrition. On top of that, we spend an estimated $60 billion a year on diet books, programs, and pills.

What do we have to show for all this effort? Not much. Americans still get nearly 35% of their calories from fat, more than is recommended as healthy. A whopping 54% of us are overweight, and more than 20% of us fall into the obese category. Adults are increasingly diagnosed with diabetes, again largely due to obesity, sedentary lifestyle, and diet. All three of these factors—fatty diet, obesity, and diabetes—contribute to heart disease, the leading cause of death among both men and women.

176

Why do people have such trouble managing their diets? As a survey by former Surgeon General C. Everett Koop shows, the message that fat is bad may be completely overshadowing an equally important message—that too many calories are just as harmful. To examine the dietary practices of overweight Americans, Dr. Koop, through his "Shape Up, America!" campaign, commissioned Louis Harris and Associates to poll 2,000 adults whose body-mass index was 25 or more. This number, remember, takes into account both an individual's weight and height, and is a good predictor of lifestyle-related disease risk. People with a body-mass index under 25 are considered to have an appropriate weight for their height, while those with a body-mass index of 25 or more fall into the overweight category.

To qualify for this X-FACTOR (Excessive Fat and Consumption Trends in Obesity Risk) survey, a person 5′4″ had to weigh at least 150 pounds, and a 5′10″ individual had to weigh 175 pounds or more. Among those who took part in the survey, the women averaged 5′4″ and 175 pounds, and the men averaged 5′10″ and 203 pounds. According to this poll:

- Among overweight Americans, 78% are not currently dieting. Even among people at very high risk, only 37% said they were dieting to lose weight. This may reflect a lack of understanding about the relationship between obesity and poor health. Most of those polled said they were aware that they should reduce dietary fat, even if they didn't know how to put this recommendation into practice, with 67% recognizing the cause-and-effect relationship between limiting fat intake and good health.
- Less than half of the respondents (42%) said they were trying to limit their intake of calories, even though the only way to lose weight is by limiting calories and exercising.
- Among those who said they were dieting, the most popular strategy was trying to limit the amount of fat in the diet (89% were trying this) while fewer people (71%) were also trying to limit the number of calories they consumed.

If the X-FACTOR poll is an accurate indicator, many Americans don't understand that controlling calorie intake is just as important as controlling fat intake when it comes to weight management. If you want to maintain your weight, you must balance the calories—whatever their source—that you take in through your diet with the calories that are expended through physical activity. If you want to lose weight, you have to change that balance so that you're burning more calories than you're taking in.

If you have similar problems managing your diet, take heart. In this chapter, we'll show you how minor adjustments in your eating habits can have a tremendous effect on your weight over time. In addition, we will:

- Talk about the dangers of obesity
- Show how minor changes in your diet and exercise routines can have a major effect on your weight over time
- Offer highlights of the American Heart Association's Dietary Guidelines for Healthy American Adults
- Include a food diary you can fill out to help you become aware of what you're eating and how you are feeling when you choose to eat (see Box 48)
- Discuss the importance of portion control, and review how much one serving is
- Highlight common eating mistakes that can add extra pounds
- Point out that your motivation for exercise—or lack of it—on any given day is more than a matter of self-discipline; it also has much to do with what you ate during the day and when you ate it

The Dangers of Being Overweight

What causes a person to become overweight or obese? There's no single easy-to-identify and easy-to-change cause. Research has shown that excess weight stems from a number of factors, including your genetic makeup and your lifestyle choices. So while it would be misleading to conclude that inactivity *is the only cause* of weighing too much, it is accurate to say that it results from taking in more calories than you burn. It follows, then, that burning more calories through regular, moderate exercise is likely to result in a healthy body weight—providing of course that you eat a moderate diet.

BOX 48

Daily Food Diary

Date					
Meal	Time	Mood	Hunger level	Foods	Calories
Breakfast					
Morning snack					
Lunch					
Afternoon snack					
Dinner					
Evening snack					
		Total calories for the day			

The further you stray beyond a healthy weight during adulthood, the higher your chances of developing a variety of diseases and medical conditions. Too much weight has been associated with heart disease, stroke, high blood pressure, and high levels of hazardous LDL cholesterol. Overweight women have a higher chance of developing cancer of the gallbladder, liver, breast, uterus, and ovary. Excess weight dramatically increases a person's risk of developing diabetes and puts undue stress on muscles and joints, leading to joint and back problems. It also increases risks during pregnancy.

In the Framingham Heart Study, for example, weight gain was associated with increases in systolic blood pressure and in levels of serum glucose and serum cholesterol, which lead to a 30% to 40% increased incidence of heart disease. Weighing too much also shortens lives. The Nurses' Health Study found a direct connection between weight and mortality. Over a 16-year-period, among the more than 115,000 nurses who volunteered for this study, those who were mildly overweight died in higher numbers than those who were not, and the most overweight women—those with a body-mass index of 32 or higher—were four times more likely to die of heart disease and twice as likely to die of cancer.

The Nurses' Health Study also showed that weight gain is an independent predictor of type 2 diabetes. Why? Extra weight is mostly fat. Fatty tissue does not use insulin efficiently, causing an increase in blood sugar. This, in turn, signals the pancreas to produce more insulin, which then builds up in the blood for a while before dropping to normal, or below normal, levels. This vicious cycle is the hallmark of type 2 diabetes (also called adult-onset diabetes or non-insulin-dependent diabetes). The combination of high glucose and high insulin can cause high blood pressure and elevate levels of potentially harmful LDL cholesterol.

Exercise helps cells use blood glucose more efficiently. It also builds muscle, which is far better at using glucose than fat. This one-two combination offers potent protection against type 2 diabetes and also helps people with this condition control their blood sugar. A 1994 study of 6,000 University of Pennsylvania alumni, for example, found that every 2,000 calories of energy expended in leisure-time physical activity per week reduced by 24% the risk of developing type 2 diabetes, and even more among those at high risk for developing this disease. Results from the Nurses' Health Study also showed that exercise reduces the risk of developing type 2 diabetes.

Where You Carry Extra Weight Also Matters

A number of studies have shown a relationship between weight accumulated in the chest and waist area and an increased risk of heart disease. For some reason, blood cholesterol levels are influenced by where fat is deposited. People who carry most of their fat around the waist, for example, have lower levels of HDL (good) cholesterol than people who carry most of their fat around the hips. The Nurse's Health Study has also shown a relationship between waist-to-hip circumference and heart disease. Women whose waist-to-hip ratio was 0.88 (meaning that their waist measurement was equal to 88% of their hip measurement) or higher were three times more likely to have a heart attack or die of heart disease than women with a waist-to-hip ratio of 0.72 or lower.

You can't do anything to affect where you'll put on fat when you start gaining weight. Nor can you *specifically* control where fat will gradually melt away as you exercise and eat a better diet. But researchers from Washington University in St. Louis have shown that moderate activity can help redistribute body fat. They asked sedentary 60- to 70-year-old men and women to jog or walk briskly an average of four times a week for 45 minutes at a time. Within 9 to 12 months, these newly active individuals had lost up to 1½ inches from their waists. Over the same period, their blood cholesterol levels fell from an average of 205 mg/dl to 194, and their triglyceride levels fell from 156 to 124 mg/dl. Blood sugar levels dropped dramatically too, decreasing their risk of complications from diabetes.

Diet also makes a difference in weight distribution. Researchers at the American Cancer Society who followed 80,000 middle-aged individuals for 10 years found that those who ate at least 19 servings of vegetables each week (about 3 servings per day) were significantly less likely to gain weight around the middle than people who ate fewer vegetables. Conversely, those who ate more than three servings of red meat each week were *more* likely to gain weight around their waists.

Moderate Changes in Diet and Exercise Are Best

While we encourage you to monitor your consumption of calories and fat, we would like to caution you against making extreme changes in your diet. No matter how much weight you might want to lose, you still need a minimum of 1,200 to 1,500 calories per day, and at least 20% of those calories should come from fat. Helen, a 26-year-old who lost 65 pounds in four months through a spartan diet and vigorous exercise, learned about the dangers of a too-restrictive diet the hard way—her rapid weight loss caused her to develop gallstones. "I was 175 and got down to 130 in 4½ months. It was great to lose the weight, but long term, the diet I was on was not realistic. You can't eat 1,000 calories a day without health problems. I developed gallstones and nearly had to have surgery. I went on medication for six months, and my gallstones are gone right now. It would have been better for me to have lost the weight more slowly. I now eat about 1,500 calories and 33 to 35 fat grams a day, and I exercise—aerobics and weights. While the number of calories I eat is still on the low end, I have more energy."

Moderate changes are best for activity as well. As pointed out in Chapter 3, just one half hour of moderate exercise each day, such as a brisk, 30-minute walk that burns 150 calories, can make a difference in your weight over the long term. Let's assume that you walk for 30 minutes a day, five days a week, for one year. If your diet remained unchanged, you could lose a shade over 11 pounds (150 calories × 260 days ÷ 3,500 calories per pound = 11.14 pounds).

Now, let's say you *also* cut 200 calories from your daily diet by eliminating your bedtime snack. That's another 20 pounds (200 calories × 365 days ÷ 3,500 calories per pound = 20.9 pounds).

As you can see, this simple combination of walking five days a week and moderate calorie restriction every day could help you lose 30 pounds over the course of a year. And don't forget the other benefits—extra energy, better mood, improved self-esteem, all of which could further motivate you to exercise and watch your diet.

Of course, the reverse is also true. If you start *adding* a snack at night to your diet on a regular basis, and you were to burn 150 fewer calories per day due to inactivity, you could just as easily *gain* 30 pounds over a year.

Dietary Guidelines for Americans

Beginning in 1980, the government began publishing nutritional guidelines aimed at helping people eat for health as much as for hunger and pleasure. Since then, other versions have been proffered by organizations such as the American Heart Association, American Diabetes Association, American Cancer Society, and others. All of these separate guidelines are remarkably similar, prompting the 1999 publication of a set of common guidelines backed by all these organizations. The distilled nutritional wisdom in the guidelines is simple and straightforward, sounding much like what you used to hear from your parents.

- **Eat a variety of foods:** Include fruits and vegetables, nonfat and low-fat dairy products, whole-grain breads, cereals, pastas, starchy vegetables, beans, lean meat, skinless poultry, and fish.
- **Balance the food you eat with physical activity:** If your weight is in the healthy category, striking a balance between the number of calories you take in and the number you expend will keep you there. If you weigh more than you want to, or more than is healthy, cutting back on calories and increasing physical activity, even a little bit, will help you lose weight.
- **Choose a diet with plenty of grain products, vegetables and fruits:** These foods should contribute the majority of your daily energy intake—between 55% and 60% of total calories. Fruits, vegetables, whole grains, and legumes provide important vitamins, minerals, fiber, and complex carbohydrates. Diets high in unrefined carbohydrates also tend to be high in both soluble and insoluble fiber.
- **Choose a diet low in fat, saturated fat, and cholesterol:** The guidelines generally suggest getting no more than 30% of your calories

from fat. The amount of saturated fat in your diet strongly influences the amount of LDL (bad) cholesterol in your bloodstream, so
less than 10% of total calories should come from saturated fats such
as those found in whole-milk dairy products and fatty meat. Trans
fatty acids, found in certain margarines and shortening should also
be avoided. Polyunsaturated fats, such as those found in safflower
and other vegetable oils, or monounsaturated fats, such as those
found in olive oil or canola oil, certainly contribute calories but
aren't as bad for you as saturated fats.

- **Choose a diet moderate in sugars:** Although sugar intake has not
  been directly related to risk for cardiovascular disease, diets high in
  refined carbohydrates are often high in calories and fat and low in
  complex carbohydrates, fiber, vitamins, and minerals.
- **Choose a diet moderate in salt and sodium:** Many studies have
  shown a strong connection between salt intake and blood pressure.
  To stay on the safe side, try keeping the amount of salt you get to
  under six grams a day. Keep in mind that relatively little of this
  comes from the salt shaker on your table; most comes from prepared foods.
- **If you drink alcoholic beverages, do so in moderation:** Drinking in
  excess is a leading cause of preventable death and disease. That
  said, there is some evidence that drinking moderate amounts of alcohol, roughly defined as a drink a day (5 ounces of wine, 12 ounces
  of beer, or 1.5 ounces of 80-proof liquor), may offer some protection against heart disease in both men and women.

These guidelines, which are meant to apply to everyone two years
of age and older, represent a consensus of the nation's health and nutrition organizations about the role of diet in reducing the risk of lifestyle-related disease. The newest guidelines emphasize exercise more
than previous versions did, acknowledging that physical activity is
important to weight control, as well as to immune function and overall health.

A graphic representation of these guidelines is the Food Guide
Pyramid introduced by the U.S. Department of Agriculture and the
Department of Health and Human Services in 1992. It illustrates the
combination and proportion of the foods you need for a healthy diet,

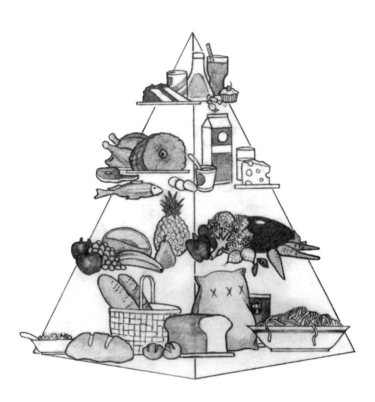

striking a balance between variety and reduced fat. The idea is to eat more servings from the groups at the *bottom* of the pyramid (breads, cereals, rice, and pasta) and fewer from the top level (fats, oils, and sweets). While 6 to 11 servings of breads, cereals, and pasta may seem like a lot of food, keep in mind that serving sizes are quite small (see Box 49). Also note that the pyramid suggests *a range of recommended servings* from each group that is determined by your age, gender, and level of physical activity. For example, a sedentary women may need only 6 servings from the grain group while a very active woman may need the full 11 (see Box 50).

If you have gained weight over time, one of the reasons may be because the portions you consume are too generous. For example, a single serving of meat, poultry, or fish is three ounces—the size of a deck of cards. If portion control is a problem to you, consider buying an inexpensive food scale, and then use it!

BOX 49

What Counts as a Serving?

Bread, cereal, rice, pasta	1 slice of bread	1 ounce ready-to-eat cereal	½ cup cooked cereal, rice, or pasta
Vegetables	1 cup raw leafy vegetables	½ cup other vegetables, cooked or chopped raw	¾ cup vegetable juice
Fruit	1 medium apple, banana, pear, orange	½ cup chopped, cooked, or canned fruit	¾ cup fruit juice
Milk, yogurt, cheese	1 cup milk or yogurt	1 ½ ounces natural cheese	2 ounces processed cheese
Meat, poultry, fish, dry beans, eggs, and nuts	2–3 ounces cooked lean meat, poultry, or fish	½ cup cooked dry beans or 1 egg equals 1 ounce cooked lean meat	2 tablespoons peanut butter or 1/3 cup nuts equals 1 ounce cooked lean meat

Interpreting Food Labels

Once upon a time, making intelligent choices in the grocery store was next to impossible. There was little uniformity in food labeling, and comparing food products was difficult. Manufacturers had free reign when it came to product claims, so it was hard to know what to believe. Enter the Nutrition Labeling and Education Act of 1990, which standardized serving sizes and required ingredients to be listed in descending order by weight. The new labels also help you budget your calories, fat, saturated fat, cholesterol, sodium, carbohydrates, and vitamins for the day. Using the expression "percentage daily value," the label lists how much of a particular nutrient this particular food gives you of the amount required for your daily diet. This replaces the old "recommended daily allowances" (RDA) method you may be more familiar with. In addition, the 1990 act requires that product claims such as "low fat" or "high fiber" must be truthful.

When considering daily values, remember that they are related to the serving size listed on the package. If the serving size is one cup and you eat two cups, the percentage daily value doubles as well. It's also important to consider that daily values are based on a 2,000 calorie diet, which is appropriate for moderately active women, sedentary men, and teenage girls. If your goal is weight loss and you plan to

BOX 50

Sample Daily Diets at Three Calorie Levels

Food group	1,600 calories	2,200 calories	2,800 calories
Grain (servings)	6	9	11
Vegetables (servings)	3	4	5
Fruit (servings)	2	3	4
Milk products (servings)	2–3	2–3	2–3
Meat (ounces)	5	6	7
Total fat (grams)	53	73	93
Total added sugars (teaspoons)	6	12	18

eat less than 2,000 calories per day, be sure to consult a nutritionist to determine if your calorie intake is appropriate for your goals and your health, and how you need to adjust your percentage daily values at your calorie-intake level.

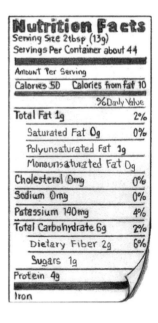

Serving sizes are based on a typical portion as determined by U.S. government surveys. All other information on the label relates to this measure. The amounts per serving—the numbers listed next to the nutrients listed—show how much of each nutrient a serving contains. According to the labeling law, labels must list serving size, number of servings per container, and amount of the following in each serving: total calories, total calories from fat, total fat, saturated fat, cholesterol, sodium, total carbohydrates, complex carbohydrates, sugars, dietary fiber, and total protein. Values for other vitamins or minerals will be listed if the product package makes a claim for them. Finally, the labels list the recommended total daily amounts of the key nutrients, in milligrams or grams, for both 2,000 and 2,500 calorie daily diets.

Do You Need Supplements?

The media has made much of the supposed benefits of the antioxidant vitamins A, C, and E and their potential link to lower rates of heart disease, cancer, diabetes, and age-related eye diseases like cataract. At this point, though, we just don't know if these vitamins actually protect people from heart disease or if people who take vitamins also do other things (such as exercise, eat healthier, or see their physicians more often) that might be what are really protecting them from heart disease. Because the jury is still out on these antioxidant vitamins, the American Heart Association and other groups suggest that people eat plenty of vitamin-rich fruits and vegetables.

Folic acid and vitamins B_6 and B_{12} have also been receiving a lot of attention in recent years. Folic acid is crucial to fetal development soon after conception. Too little of this B vitamin early in pregnancy may prevent a fetus's spinal cord and spine from developing as they should. The result could be the serious birth defects called spina bifida or anencephaly (the latter is always fatal). That's the main reason why all women in their child-bearing years are urged to get at least 400 micrograms of folic acid a day.

Folic acid, along with vitamins B_6 and B_{12}, can also lower levels of a substance in the blood called homocysteine, which comes from the breakdown of protein. High blood levels of homocysteine have been linked with coronary heart disease, stroke, and circulation problems in the arms, legs, and other parts of the body. A number of studies show that men and women who get lots of folate, vitamin B_6, and vitamin B_{12}—and so have lower levels of homocysteine—are less likely to have heart attacks. So far, though, no completed clinical trials have tested whether reducing homocysteine levels by taking supplements of folic acid or of vitamins B_6 or B_{12} protects against heart disease or other circulation problems.

Another possible benefit of plenty of folic acid may be a lower risk of colon cancer. In the Nurses' Health Study, women who took a daily multivitamin for 15 years developed colon cancer at much lower rates than those who did not take a multivitamin. The ingredient most likely to account for this is folic acid, which has been linked with lower rates of colon cancer in several studies.

The only supplements (aside from folic acid) that do have widespread support for a particular group of women are calcium and vitamin D supplements for postmenopausal women. These may help preserve bone mass. The latest recommendation for calcium intake among women aged 19 to 50 is 1,000 milligrams of calcium a day, and for postmenopausal women 1,200–1,500 milligrams a day. The recommendation for vitamin D is 400–600 IU daily.

Eating Well for Exercise

You need energy to exercise. Food is an energy source. Ergo, if you don't eat properly during the day, you may not have the physical energy or the mental drive to exercise. It's a matter of common sense. Following these simple suggestions for how much and when to eat may make sticking with your exercise program much easier.

- **Eat breakfast:** Skip this important meal and you may find yourself running out of steam partway through the morning, physically sluggish and not as mentally sharp as you'd like. Skipping breakfast may also tempt you to have that high-fat donut during a mid-morning meeting, or some butter cookies with your kids. Or you might be so hungry at lunch that you eat an extra-large portion. As a rule, it's a good idea to find ways to keep from becoming too hungry at any time, because in that state you'll be tempted to choose any food that's available. And as you well know, available food is usually fast food, which tends to be high in fat, salt, and sugar and low in nutrition.
- **Don't skip meals:** While many people think this is a good way to lose weight, just the opposite is true. When you skip a meal, your metabolism slows down a bit. A better strategy is to eat a small, nourishing snack.
- **Graze:** While most of us are conditioned to eat three meals at appointed times, our bodies may require something different. Grazing—something that strong, lean animals do—requires eating four or five small meals when you feel hunger rather than three large ones morning, noon, and evening. Learn to carry a "grazing survival pack" with you that consists of bananas, low-fat whole-wheat pretzels, nonfat yogurt, juice, and other wholesome foods. That way, you won't grab the first food you see because you're too hungry. (For other ways to avoid eating extra calories, see Box 51.)
- **Include adequate protein in your diet:** Poultry and fish are excellent sources of protein, as are lean red meats. If you are a vegetarian, you can get protein from beans, tofu, hummus, peanuts, peanut butter, nuts, and (if your diet allows them) eggs, cheese, yogurt, and other dairy products.
- **Snack before you exercise:** It's 5 P.M., you're finishing work, and you're planning to walk for 30 minutes when you get home. But you're mentally and physically tired, and hungry to boot. Exercise is the last thing you want to do, and heading for the couch as soon as you get through your front door is the first thing. What to do? An hour before you walk, have a healthy snack from your survival pack. Chances are, you'll feel much more like walking when you get home due to the energy boost you get from your snack.

• **Drink enough fluid:** Your body requires plenty of water to have an adequate supply for your blood, sweat, and tears. Water aids digestion and other important bodily functions as well. You've probably heard that you need to drink 8 eight-ounce glasses of water a day to keep yourself properly hydrated, and more if you've been active or exercising. That's not exactly true. For one thing, almost any beverage contributes to your water balance. (Those containing caffeine or alcohol don't, because these substances increase the amount of water you excrete.) Plain water is best, though, because it gives you the fluid you need without any empty calories. For another, everyone is different in the exact amount of fluid needed each day. Unfortunately, thirst isn't a perfect signal that you need something to drink, especially among older people, who may not feel thirsty as

BOX 51

Simple Tricks for Avoiding Extra Calories

• Don't snack while you cook, drive, or watch TV or movies.
• Don't finish those leftovers or foods the kids don't eat; freeze them or throw them out.
• Avoid fried foods and sugary drinks.
• Choose skinless chicken and fish over red meat.
• Limit portion sizes.
• Choose light, low-fat salad dressings and use them on the side.
• Choose fruit for snacks or dessert, rather than baked goods or ice cream.
• Try jam on your toast instead of butter or margarine.
• Buy 1% milk and then gradually acclimate your taste buds (and eyes) to skim, by mixing 1% with skim.
• In restaurants, skip the bread, butter, and appetizer; or order an appetizer with a salad instead of an entrée.
• For portion control when eating out, split an entrée with someone in your party, or take half of it home with you.

often as they "should." Other indicators can be tipoffs that you aren't getting enough fluid. Deep yellow or brownish urine is a sure sign that you need more water, while pale yellow urine is a sign that you're drinking enough. If you regularly wake up feeling tired, groggy, and headachy despite enough sleep, too little water may be the culprit.

Avoid the "Work It Off" Trap

Another mistake that many people make is overeating and then trying to burn those excess calories off with exercise. This approach turns exercise into punishment instead of a healthy, enjoyable activity. Why cheat yourself out of the pleasure of a brisk walk on a beautiful day by pushing yourself to jog until you're exhausted? In addition, it takes a lot more exercise to burn off food than you think. For example, one tablespoon of butter has about 100 calories. If you weigh 150 pounds, it can take as much as one mile of running or two miles of brisk walking to burn off that small amount of butter.

But don't let this seemingly unfair imbalance between pleasure and work prompt you to give up on exercise. While your workout may not burn off as many calories as you'd like as quickly as you'd like, physical activity does keep your metabolic rate up for some time after you slow down. It also helps to maintain muscle mass, which keeps your metabolism humming. When your metabolism is stoked, you burn more calories with everything you do.

Points to Remember

- Being overweight results from a number of factors, including genetic makeup and lifestyle choices, so it's not accurate to conclude that inactivity is the only cause of excess weight.
- Excess weight and obesity have been associated with heart disease, stroke, high blood pressure, and high levels of LDL (bad) cholesterol and triglycerides. Women who are overweight have a higher chance of developing cancer of the gallbladder, liver, breast, uterus, ovary, and colon. They are also at increased risk of developing type 2 diabetes, osteoarthritis, and joint and back problems.

- Small changes in diet and exercise will make a difference in your weight over time.
- On a daily basis, eating well for exercise can help you have the energy you need for your workout. Eat breakfast, don't skip meals, include adequate protein in your diet, drink plenty of fluids, eat small meals during the day, and enjoy a healthy snack an hour before your workout.

11

The Scientific Case for Physical Activity

In earlier chapters we highlighted the benefits of physical activity and exercise. Now we would like to lay out some of the detailed scientific evidence that fuels our enthusiasm and supports why we firmly believe that despite all the major technological advances in medicine, *there is probably nothing you can do that will improve your health more than being physically active.* Even if we have already managed to convince you of this, breezing through this chapter may give you extra motivation to get moving and stay active.

Measuring the Benefits of Exercise

Although it may be hard to believe, identifying and quantifying the benefits of physical activity is a daunting challenge. Why? Because studying *anything* in humans is a challenge. One of the keys to good science is tight control, something scientists do not have—and should not have—when working with humans. Say, for example, that a research team wanted to investigate the effect of 30 minutes of daily moderate activity on the development of diabetes. The ideal way to determine this would be to assemble many people, divide them into two groups, and then make sure that the only thing different between the groups was that the members of one did 30 minutes of exercise each day and the members of the other *absolutely did not exercise.* Everyone participating in the study would need to eat the same diet,

194

work similar types of jobs, face similar stresses, and so on, for ten years or more—long enough for a significant number of cases of diabetes to be diagnosed. Such a study would be thoroughly unethical, as well as logistically and financially impractical.

In place of this type of "decisive" study, we must rely on evidence that comes from less definitive kinds of research, each with its own strengths and limitations. The remarkable thing is that the evidence from all different types of studies, in different populations, points in the same direction—toward the benefits of physical activity.

There is a vast amount of information from highly controlled animal studies showing, without a doubt, that physical activity improves health and lengthens the life span. The results from such studies only point to the possibilities that exist for us humans. The four main types of human studies are:

- **Cross-sectional studies:** These are "snapshots" of a population at a moment in time. They usually take the form of surveys that assess things like exercise, diet, and health.
- **Case-control studies:** These studies are a kind of "look back" investigation. Researchers assemble a group of cases—people with a particular disease or condition, such as breast cancer or heart disease. For each case, they also find one or two people who are similar in age and sex but who do not have the disease. Then the investigators compare the two groups, looking for differences in diets, habits, medical histories, or whatever.
- **Cohort studies:** Cohort studies are more a kind of "look forward" investigation. Researchers assemble a group of individuals—nurses in the case of the Nurses' Health Study, women living in several counties in Iowa in the case of the Iowa Women's Health Study—gather as much information about them as possible, then follow their health over as long a time period as possible.
- **Randomized trials:** In randomized trials, volunteers are assigned to an "intervention," such as exercising several times a week, or to a control group with no formal exercise program, and then differences in the health of the two groups are compared some years down the road.

No single study will ever offer definite proof that moderate exercise is *the best route* to better health. But consistent evidence from all four types of study, plus compelling evidence from animal studies, clearly underscores the importance of moderate activity in maintaining health and preventing chronic disease.

In the following sections, we will lay down the scientific underpinning of this book. Not all of it, of course—that would require a textbook. Instead, we will point out some of the highlights of research

BOX 52

Quantifying the Health Benefits of Exercise

↓ Premature death	30% to 50% reduced risk
↓ Heart disease	40% to 50% reduced risk
↓ Stroke	30% to 50% reduced risk
↓ Blood pressure	Lowers blood pressure
↓ Cholesterol	Lowers LDL and triglycerides Raises HDL
↓ Obesity	Helps with weight reduction Reduces abdominal and total fat Increases metabolism and muscle mass
↓ Type 2 (adult-onset) diabetes	30% to 40% reduced risk Improves blood sugar control
↓ Breast cancer	20% to 30% reduced risk
↓ Colon cancer	30% to 50% reduced risk
↓ Osteoporosis	40% to 50% reduced risk of a broken hip
↓ Depression/stress	Relieves stress Improves mood
↑ Emotional well-being	Increases energy level Improves outlook on life

into the connection between lack of physical activity and early death, heart disease, stroke, high cholesterol, high blood pressure, diabetes, obesity, distribution of body fat, cancer, bone loss, and poor balance in old age (see Box 52).

Increased Longevity

The inescapable conclusion from studies of physical activity is that if you want to live longer, and live more of those years free of chronic disease, start exercising today and stay active for the rest of your life. One of the most consistent findings is that *increasing levels of exercise are associated with decreasing mortality rates.* In plain English, this means that in studies of exercise, a smaller percentage of people in the exercise group died during the study period than in the non-exercise group. It also means that the greater the intensity and duration of exercise, the lower the death rate. (This isn't due to the fact that people who already had underlying illness were just too sick to exercise—most studies exclude people with health problems that limit their activity.) Keep in mind that these are results for *populations,* not individuals. In each study, some people who exercised died, and some who did not exercise didn't die. So there's no way to predict with great accuracy whether you, or any individual, will live a long and healthy life if you exercise. But the odds are on your side if you choose to start.

- Several important studies have come from the Cooper Institute for Aerobics Research in Dallas. One of these found that low levels of physical fitness increased the odds of dying from all causes for both men and women. Among the 3,120 women in the eight-year study, the death rate dropped from 39.5 per 10,000 person-years among the least active group to 8.5 among the most active group; for men, the rates dropped from 64 per 10,000 person-years to 18.6. The lower death rate in the most active group was mostly due to fewer deaths from heart disease and cancer (see Box 53).
- Two other Cooper Institute for Aerobics Research studies of note: A 1995 report on almost 10,000 men followed for five years showed that it's never too late to start reaping benefits from exercise. The

death rate in the group of men who were the least physically fit for the entire period was three times higher than that for the most fit men. The men who made a shift from an inactive lifestyle to an active one during the study period reduced their risk of dying by almost half. A 1996 study of 32,000 men and women showed that the protective effect of exercise applied even to people who smoked and who had high blood pressure and high cholesterol. Physically active smokers were less likely to have died over the study period than inactive smokers.

• A study of more than 10,000 men who graduated from Harvard University and who answered several health questionnaires between 1962 and 1985 revealed four important ways to lower the

BOX 53

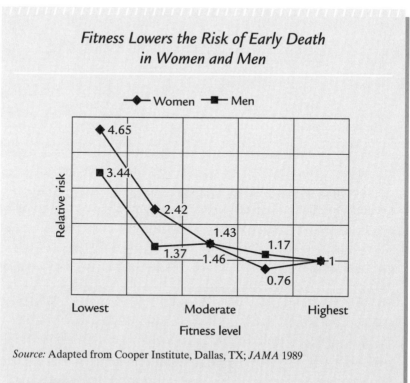

Fitness Lowers the Risk of Early Death in Women and Men

—◆— Women —■— Men

4.65

3.44

2.42

1.43

1.17

1.37

1.46

0.76

1

Relative risk

Lowest   Moderate   Highest

Fitness level

Source: Adapted from Cooper Institute, Dallas, TX; *JAMA* 1989

chances of dying prematurely: (1) begin some kind of moderately vigorous activity such as brisk walking, (2) stop smoking, (3) keep blood pressure in the normal range, and (4) don't gain weight. The men who became more active between answering the first and second questionnaires were 23% less likely to have died than their counterparts who remained inactive during this period.

- The more energy these Harvard alums expended in exercise, the lower their chances of dying. In other words, there was a dose-response relationship between physical activity and mortality. In addition, moderate exercise improved cholesterol levels and the body's ability to use glucose. Men who became active even in middle age extended their lives by nearly a year, compared with those who remained sedentary. Extra years of life were seen with increased physical activity in all age groups, even above age 75.

- The Iowa Women's Health Study tracked more than 40,000 post-menopausal women for seven years. A smaller proportion of the women who reported they were physically active died during the study than the inactive women. As with the Harvard alums, the more the Iowa women exercised, the less likely they were to die during the follow-up period.

- A 20-year Swedish study of 1,400 initially healthy women showed that women who had low levels of physical activity at the beginning of the study, as well as those who decreased their physical activity during the study, were more likely to have died during the 20-year follow-up period than those women who were initially active or who became more active during that period.

- We tend to blame a lot of things on our genes, but a key study of identical twins living in Finland shows that physical activity may play as large a role as heredity in determining how long we live. Researchers followed 7,500 pairs of identical twins for 19 years. In cases where the two twins' activity levels differed markedly from each other, the twin who exercised at least 6 times a month for 30 minutes was half as likely to have died during the study period as the twin who was inactive. The inescapable conclusion from these twins studies is that physical activity contributes significantly to longevity.

- The Cardiovascular Health Study was designed to look at factors contributing to death and illness among people between the ages of 65 and 101. The average age of the 5,201 participants was 73. The least active participants were the most likely to have died during the five-year study. Increasing amounts of exercise decreased the chances of dying. The researchers estimated that taking a 30-minute walk five times a week could cut one's risk of dying in half.
- Must exercise be vigorous to prevent premature death? Not according to the Honolulu Heart Program, which has followed more than 8,000 men of Japanese ancestry living on the island of Oahu since 1965. This study included 707 nonsmoking retired men between the ages of 61 and 81 who answered questionnaires on walking in 1980 and 1982. Over the next 12 years, the death rate among the men who walked less than one mile per day was nearly twice that for those who walked more than two miles per day, indicating that regular walking confers benefits.

Heart Disease and Stroke

The latest numbers from the National Center for Health Statistics show that heart disease and stroke account for 40% of all deaths in the United States. That's as true for women as it is for men. Actually, more women than men die each year from heart disease and stroke, and *these two diseases claim more women's lives than the next 16 causes of death combined!* In other words, breast cancer and cancers of the colon, lung, and reproductive system are not nearly as threatening to the lives of women as are heart disease and stroke. The good news is that regular physical activity decreases your risk of developing or dying from heart disease, especially from heart attacks caused by clogged coronary arteries. In fact, becoming physically active *is as important to the health of your heart as quitting smoking.*

There is also mounting evidence that exercise prevents stroke, although this link isn't as conclusive as the link between physical activity and heart disease. Prevention is particularly important for this disease because treatment options are usually quite limited after a stroke has occurred. Numerous studies indicate that, as with exercise

and premature death, the benefit derived from physical activity occurs even with moderate levels of fitness, and it increases as the
fitness level increases.

HEART DISEASE

- One of the pre-eminent studies of heart disease in America is the
  Framingham Heart Study, which since 1948 has tracked the health,
  habits, and illnesses of more than 5,000 men and women in a single Massachusetts town. After 24 years, women in the study with inactive lifestyles were 2.5 times more likely to have had a heart attack or to develop some other form of coronary heart disease than
  women who were active.
- The Cooper Institute for Aerobics Research in Dallas and the Harvard Alumni Study each found strong inverse relationships between
  physical fitness and death from cardiovascular disease. The Institute reported that women in the lowest ranking of physical fitness
  had a death rate from cardiovascular disease of 7.4 per 10,000 person-years over an eight-year study period, compared with 2.9 for
  women in the middle ranking and 0.8 for women in the top category
  of physical fitness. The Harvard Alumni Study showed that regular
  post-college exercise, not in-college sports play, offered some protection against heart attacks and coronary heart disease. Ex-ath-
  letes who became sedentary were far more likely to face these medical conditions than sedentary students who became active later
  in life.
- When researchers studied 17,000 female Seventh-Day Adventists,
  a population with a relatively low risk for cardiovascular disease,
  they found that a higher level of physical activity was strongly related with a lower chance of dying from heart disease.
- The ongoing Nurses' Health Study at Harvard's Brigham and
  Women's Hospital in Boston has been following more than 120,000
  female nurses since 1976. A 1999 analysis that involved almost
  73,000 of these women found that moderate physical activity such
  as brisk walking was associated with a lower heart attack risk.
  Those participants who walked at least 3 hours per week at a pace

of 3 miles an hour or faster had a 34% lower risk of developing heart disease than those who rarely exercised. Women who were sedentary at the start of the study and later became more physically active had a lower risk of heart attack than women who remained sedentary (see Box 54).

- Researchers from the University of Washington in Seattle looked at levels of physical activity among 268 postmenopausal women who had suffered heart attacks and then compared them with 925 women of similar ages who had not. The results suggest that the risk of having a heart attack is decreased 50% by 30 to 45 minutes of brisk walking three times a week, or its energy equivalent.

STROKE

Several large studies using different scientific methods show that exercise can help prevent strokes. This may be due to exercise's ability to lower weight, blood pressure, and blood sugar levels, three factors involved in triggering strokes.

BOX 54

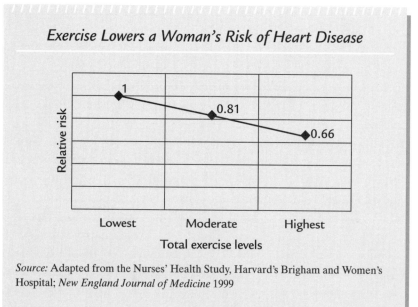

Exercise Lowers a Woman's Risk of Heart Disease

Relative risk — Total exercise levels: Lowest (1), Moderate (0.81), Highest (0.66)

Source: Adapted from the Nurses' Health Study, Harvard's Brigham and Women's Hospital; *New England Journal of Medicine* 1999

- In the late 1980s, researchers with the National Center for Health Statistics examined the health records of almost 8,000 people who had participated in the first National Health and Nutrition Examination Survey back in the early 1970s. Among men and women, blacks and whites, those who said during the interview part of the survey that they were not physically active were almost twice as likely as the more-active people to have a stroke over the next 12 years.

- A recent study of a very diverse urban population showed much the same thing. In the Northern Manhattan Stroke Study, leisure-time physical activity was clearly connected with a reduction in strokes among women and men, in younger and older groups, and among African Americans, whites, and Hispanics. In this study as in many others, the amount and intensity of exercise made a difference, with longer and more intense activity providing somewhat more protection than shorter and more moderate activity. But light-to-moderate activity and less than two hours of activity a week were far better than no activity.

High Blood Pressure and High Cholesterol

High blood pressure, also called hypertension, and high levels of cholesterol in the bloodstream are two of the most prevalent and powerful contributors to heart disease and stroke. For example, a 7 point increase in blood pressure is associated with a 27% increase in risk of coronary heart disease and a 42% increase in risk of stroke. The numbers for cholesterol are similar—for every 10% increase in total cholesterol, the risk of coronary heart disease increases 20–30%. Regular, moderate exercise can prevent the development of high blood pressure as well as reduce elevated blood pressure. It has also been shown to lower levels of LDL (bad) cholesterol and increase levels of HDL (good) cholesterol.

- The University of Pittsburgh's Healthy Women Study was designed to investigate how risk factors for cardiovascular disease change with "the change." Among the 541 premenopausal women who volunteered for this study, the women who fell into the more active groups had lower blood pressures, lower resting heart rates, lower levels of LDL (bad) cholesterol, and higher levels of HDL (good) cholesterol. The greater the activity level, the greater the improvement. After three years, average weight, blood pressure, and LDL cholesterol levels all increased, while HDL levels decreased. However, the women who reported higher levels of activity at the outset of the study had the smallest increases in weight and the smallest decreases in HDL levels.

- In the German Cardiovascular Prevention Study, almost 10,000 men and women aged 50 to 69 were followed for seven years. The greater the weekly energy expenditure, the lower the blood pressure. Among the 5,885 women, those who engaged in moderate physical activity for 30 minutes five times a week had significantly lower blood pressure and resting heart rates than their sedentary counterparts. They were also 60% less likely to have multiple risk factors for cardiovascular disease.

- In the appropriately named SWEAT (Sedentary Women Exercise Adherence Trial) study, resting blood pressure declined among 60 sedentary women who began exercising three times a week but increased among 30 women who did not begin exercising. The decreases in blood pressure weren't linked to changes in cardiovascular fitness or body weight.

- As we have been saying throughout this book, the benefits of exercise aren't reserved just for young people. In an Australian experiment involving 38 healthy women in their 80s, a twice weekly walking program lowered blood pressure and heart rates while at the same time improving daily activity patterns.

- Exercise is one way to reduce blood pressure without resorting to medications. It is among the first-line strategies recommended by the Joint National Committee on Detection, Evaluation, and Treatment of High Blood Pressure. The committee's latest guidelines recommend moderately intense physical activity, "such as 30 to 45 minutes of brisk walking most days of the week."

- A study from the University of Colorado at Boulder showed that exercise helped postmenopausal women with true hypertension (systolic blood pressure above 140 and diastolic pressure above 90) as well as those with high-normal pressures. Twelve weeks of moderate-intensity walking decreased resting blood pressure in every volunteer. On average, those with true high blood pressure were able to bring their pressures down into the high-normal range, while those who started the experiment with high-normal blood pressures ended with pressures in the mid-normal range.

- If you are taking high blood pressure medication, physical activity may help you reduce your need for it. A recent Veterans Affairs study looked at 46 African-American men who were taking medication to reduce their very high blood pressures. Half of the volunteers were assigned to a 16-week exercise program; the rest did not exercise. Of the 14 exercise patients who finished the study, 10 were able to take a reduced dosage of medication. On the average, the dosages for the entire group were lowered by about one-third. By comparison, none of the patients in the non-exercise group tolerated lower doses.

- High levels of total cholesterol and LDL (bad) cholesterol, as well as low levels of HDL (good) cholesterol, point women as well as men in the direction of heart disease. Exercise offers one way to combat wayward cholesterol levels and is, in fact, the first line of treatment suggested for them. According to the expert panel that set the latest national guidelines on treating high cholesterol, "Both weight reduction and exercise not only promote reduction of cholesterol levels but have other benefits, i.e., reducing triglycerides, raising HDL-cholesterol, reducing blood pressure, and decreasing the risk for diabetes mellitus." These guidelines are based on a number of studies showing similar trends between increasing activity and favorable changes in cholesterol levels.

- At the University of Turku in Finland, researchers asked more than 100 inactive men and women to begin an exercise program. Approximately 30 minutes of moderate physical activity a day reduced levels of LDL cholesterol by 10% and increased levels of HDL cholesterol by 15% in men and 5% in women. What's more, exercise reduced the amount of LDL in the bloodstream that was vulnerable to attack by oxygen, the first of a long series of steps that leads to the development of fatty, artery-clogging plaques.

- Most of the studies linking exercise with reductions in cholesterol

have examined the effect of aerobic exercise such as brisk walking or running. Strength training offers similar benefits, as shown
by work from the Tucson VA Medical Center. Among 46 premenopausal women assigned to a strength-training program for five
months, total and LDL cholesterol levels dropped compared to
those of 42 women not assigned to exercise.

- In the Diet and Exercise for Elevated Risk trial at Stanford University, 180 men and women with high cholesterol were assigned to one
of four groups: increased physical activity; a low-fat, low-cholesterol
diet; both increased activity and the diet; and no special intervention. A low cholesterol diet alone tended to lower levels of protective HDL cholesterol (a potentially dangerous trend), while exercise alone and diet plus exercise reversed that trend. Diet alone and
exercise alone were only marginally effective at lowering levels of
LDL cholesterol, while the combination of diet and exercise was far
more effective. In addition, the researchers suggested that some
synergy between exercise and a low-fat diet "may create a physio-
logic state that is particularly beneficial to lipid metabolism."

Obesity

Here is a sampling of the rapidly growing body of research showing
the hazards of excess weight and the benefits of exercise in reducing
weight.

- In the ongoing Framingham Heart Study, after 26 years of follow-
up, the heaviest people among the 5,200 participants had, on average, higher blood pressures, cholesterol levels, and blood sugar levels than the leanest participants. They also had higher rates of heart
disease and death. Substantial weight gain after early adulthood
also increased the risk of heart disease and early death.
- In the Nurses' Health Study, after eight years of follow-up (between
1976 and 1984), those women who had gained more than 20 pounds
since age 18 were more likely to develop or die from heart disease.
Even mild to moderate weight gains (11 to 19 pounds) increased
a woman's chances of developing heart disease. By comparison,

women whose weights were stable since early adulthood, and those who weighed 10–15 percent less than the average for women of the same age, were the least likely to develop or die from heart disease during that period. After 14 years of follow-up, the study showed that women who weighed 30% more than their recommended weight for height were four times as likely to die from heart disease.

- In a study from Tufts University, women who exercised at least 30 minutes a day on five or more days a week weighed less than their non-exercising counterparts. They also had lower blood pressures, levels of cholesterol, and levels of triglyceride (another type of blood fat). The exercisers in the study gave higher marks to their health, sense of well-being, and energy levels than did the non-exercisers, and they also missed fewer days of work due to illness.

- Can exercise help if you are already overweight? You bet. For one thing, it may help you lose weight. For another, a fit person is better off than an unfit one at any weight. At the Cooper Institute for Aerobics Research, nearly 22,000 men between the ages of 30 and 83 agreed to be analyzed for body composition and take a treadmill test to determine cardiorespiratory fitness. Eight years later, 428 of the volunteers had died, 144 from heart disease. Unsurprisingly, the lowest death rates occurred among the men labeled as fit on the basis of the two tests. But even overweight men reaped benefits from exercise, with lower death rates among the overweight men who were fit than among the overweight men who were unfit. Moreover, leanness didn't cancel out the hazards of inactivity; the lean but unfit volunteers had double the risk of death as their lean, fit counterparts.

Body Fat Distribution

As we discussed in Chapter 2, fat that accumulates around your waist causes more health problems than fat that settles around your hips or thighs. Abdominal fat is more likely to cause high cholesterol and high blood pressure, heart disease, and type 2 diabetes. Fortunately, moderate exercise can help redistribute body fat and thus lower your risk of developing heart disease and diabetes.

- A study from East Carolina University's Human Performance Laboratory showed that performing moderate physical activity for 30 to 45 minutes at least three times a week reduced the amount of abdominal fat among 13 initially inactive volunteers. It also reduced levels of total cholesterol and triglyceride, increased levels of HDL (good) cholesterol, and increased the sensitivity of muscle cells to insulin.
- Strength training also helps redistribute weight. In a University of Alabama study of older women, a 16-week strength-raining program made significant progress in whittling away abdominal fat. While neither average weight nor total body fat changed, the amount of abdominal fat decreased by 10%.

Diabetes

About 16 million Americans have diabetes, although only 10 million or so know it. Most have type 2 (adult-onset) diabetes, which develops because the body's cells become resistant to insulin, the hormone that helps transport blood sugar into cells. Diabetes can have devastating complications such as blindness, kidney failure, coronary heart disease, and circulatory problems that may result in amputation, nerve problems, and premature death. Type 2 diabetes strikes more women than men, and three out of four people who have it are substantially overweight. The incidence of the disease has been soaring in the past few decades, largely due to the increased frequency of obesity and sedentary lifestyle.

- Scores of studies have linked excess weight and weight gain with type 2 diabetes. For example, the Nurses' Health Study found that the higher the body-mass index (BMI), the higher the risk of diabetes. Compared with women whose BMIs were 22 or below (equivalent to a 5'5" woman who weighs 132 pounds or less), those with BMIs of 27.0 to 28.8 were 10 times more likely to develop diabetes, and those with BMIs greater than 35 were *60 times* more likely. Weight gain or loss after age 18 also played a role. When compared to women whose weights had been stable since early adulthood, those who had gained between 11 and 17 pounds after age 18 doubled their chances of developing type 2 diabetes. Adding even more weight further increased the risk. However, women who had *lost* more than 11 pounds cut in half their chances of developing diabetes.

- A number of studies in both men and women show that physical activity can prevent type 2 diabetes. The Physicians' Health Study of 21,000 male doctors, for example, found a strong connection between exercise and lower rates of diabetes. The more these men exercised, the lower their chances of developing diabetes—once a week was good, two to four times a week was better, and five or more times a week was best. Exercise appeared to be particularly helpful for men who were overweight.

- Women benefit from exercise's diabetes-preventing effects, too. The Nurses' Health Study found that participants who exercised regularly were less likely to develop type 2 diabetes over an eight-year period than women who did not routinely exercise. Contrary to the results in the Physicians' Health Study, the benefits were the same for overweight and normal-weight women. A look at the same group of women 8 years later yielded even more encouraging results. Women who walked at a normal or brisk pace for several hours a week had a 30–40% lower risk of developing type 2 diabetes than women who didn't engage in any leisure-time physical activity. Running and more vigorous activities offered similar protection.

- The multicultural Insulin Resistance Atherosclerosis Study was started several years ago to examine the relationships between problems with insulin and the development of heart disease among almost 1,500 African-American, Hispanic, and non-Hispanic white volunteers. Those who participated in "vigorous activity" at least 5 times a week were more sensitive to the effects of insulin than were those who rarely or never engaged in vigorous activity. Higher sensitivity to insulin means better handling of blood sugar and thus a lower likelihood of developing diabetes. The researchers determined that "nonvigorous activity" also improved insulin sensitivity.

- Among African-American women, high blood pressure and insulin resistance often occur together, posing a double threat to health. A study from the University of Pittsburgh Medical Center showed that just seven days of walking or stationary cycling reduced insulin levels and improved insulin sensitivity among 12 overweight African-American women with high blood pressure. These changes occurred even though none of the women lost weight.

Cancer

We know that exercise can protect us against heart disease. Can it do the same against cancer, the leading killer of women in the United States after cardiovascular disease? While there is some evidence pointing in that direction, the jury is still out on the connection between physical activity and most forms of cancer. Some large studies have shown that, in general, cancer rates decline as the amount of physical activity goes up. Others show no clear association between exercise and cancer.

A critical missing link is *how* physical activity might suppress cancer. One possibility is that by boosting the immune system, exercise may improve the body's ability to detect and kill off cancer cells before they can begin multiplying. In the case of colon cancer, regular physical activity may help move waste products through the digestive tract more quickly, limiting the time that any cancer-causing substances are in contact with the lining of the colon. Exercise may also limit the amount of reproductive hormones such as estrogen and progesterone in the blood and thus prevent these cell-stimulating hormones from starting or maintaining breast cancer growth. Finally, exercise's ability to reduce weight and body fat could somehow play a role in cancer prevention, given that excess weight and body fat increase estrogen and other hormones and put people at risk for developing a variety of cancers.

Much more research must be done in this field before we can say for certain that exercise prevents cancer. So far, the connection seems to be strongest for breast and colon cancer.

- University of Southern California researchers interviewed 545 women age 40 and under who had been diagnosed with breast cancer and 545 women of the same ages and backgrounds who did not have breast cancer. They asked about the amount of time spent on physical activity, the number of pregnancies, use of oral contraceptives, and a variety of other factors that might affect breast cancer risk. The women who exercised for about four hours a week were less than half as likely to have developed breast cancer as those who rarely exercised. The apparent protective effect of exercise was even stronger among women who had had at least one full-term pregnancy, cutting their breast cancer risk by 75%.

- A much larger study that used a completely different method found a similar favorable connection between exercise and breast cancer. Norwegian researchers followed the health of more than 25,000 women with clinical exams and follow-up questionnaires. Women who were active during their leisure time were substantially less likely to develop breast cancer over almost 14 years of follow-up. Women whose jobs involved heavy manual labor had lower risk of breast cancer than women who worked office jobs (see Box 55). Factors other than exercise may have contributed to the large differences in breast cancer risk between these occupational groups, though.

BOX 55

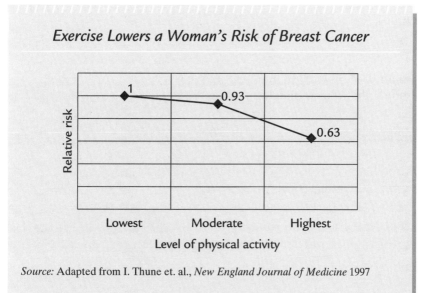

Exercise Lowers a Woman's Risk of Breast Cancer

Relative risk

1
0.93
0.63

Lowest   Moderate   Highest
Level of physical activity

Source: Adapted from I. Thune et. al., *New England Journal of Medicine* 1997

- A similar approach undertaken in the Nurses' Health Study also showed a connection between physical activity and protection against breast cancer. Women in the study reported the average number of hours they spent each week doing a variety of moderate and vigorous activities, such as walking outdoors, swimming, playing tennis, doing aerobics, or using a rowing machine. Women who spent about an hour a day doing some moderate or vigorous activity were less likely to develop breast cancer over the 16-year study period.

- Studies examining the connection between exercise and colon cancer are more consistent. A recent overview of 40 such studies estimated an average 50% reduction in colon cancer for the most active study participants compared with the least active. Colon cancer is currently the third most common type of cancer and cause of cancer death in women, after lung cancer and breast cancer. In the United States alone, each year about 95,000 people are diagnosed with colon cancer and about 48,000 die of this disease. The Harvard Medical School authors who prepared this overview estimated that increasing physical activity across all sectors of the population could decrease colon cancer by 17%, thus saving thousands of lives a year.

Osteoporosis, Broken Bones, and Other Signs of Aging

A number of scientific studies have shown that the combination of aerobic activity and strength training can delay or cancel out many of the typical signs of aging: stiffening joints, bone loss, decreased muscle tone, a slowdown in digestion, poor circulation, a slowing of reaction time, diminished short-term memory and cognitive function, sleep disorders, and depression.

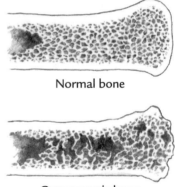

Normal bone

Osteoporotic bone

- In 1982 the Melpomene Institute, a Minneapolis research group dedicated to the study of physical activity and women's health, began examining the relationship between long-term physical activity and bone density. The ongoing study group includes 111 women initially between the ages of 46 and 80, half of whom were active at the study's start and half of whom weren't. Their health histories, diets, and levels of physical activity were logged and analyzed. A preliminary result: the women who have been engaging in physical activity throughout their lives had bone densities that were about 25% higher than those of women who had been inactive.

- The Study of Osteoporotic Fractures has followed the bone health of 9,700 women for an average of eight years. In this large group, women who were relatively inactive were the most likely to have hip fractures; those who engaged in light activities such as easy walking and gardening were less likely to fracture a hip; and those who engaged in moderately intense or vigorous activities, such as aerobic dance, tennis, or weight training, were the least likely to have hip fractures—about 45% less than the inactive women. *Any* physical activity, though, including housework, gardening, and so-

BOX 56

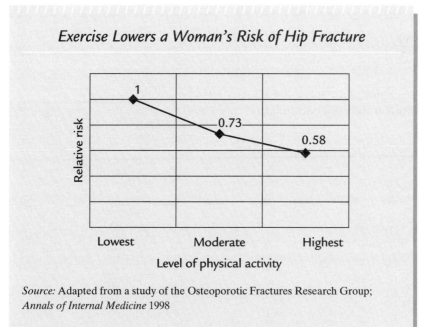

Exercise Lowers a Woman's Risk of Hip Fracture

Source: Adapted from a study of the Osteoporotic Fractures Research Group; *Annals of Internal Medicine* 1998

cial dancing, was beneficial. Looked at another way, the women who sat for more than nine hours a day had 40% more broken hips than the women who sat fewer than six hours per day (see Box 56).

- At Tufts University's USDA Human Nutrition Research Center on Aging, researchers asked 20 sedentary, older women to participate in a high-intensity strength-training program. At the end of a year, their bones had actually become more dense (and thus more sturdy), while bone density *decreased* among 20 non-exercising women who served as controls. What's more, both muscle strength and balance improved in the exercising women and decreased in the controls. Also noteworthy is that two women in the non-exercising control group fell and broke their wrists during the study, while none of the women in the exercise group suffered a fracture.

- A leading institution studying the benefits of strength training for older adults is Boston's Hebrew Rehabilitation Center for the Aged. We described one of its studies on strength training and mood in Chapter 2. Other findings suggest that strength training improves stair-climbing power, increases the level of spontaneous physical activity, and generally counteracts muscle weakness and physical frailty in older people. Another very practical finding from this center is that 8 weeks of strength training among a group of 10 men and women ranging in age from 87 to 96 shortened the time it took to walk a distance of 20 feet, the approximate width of a typical city street.

Points to Remember

- Exercise can literally add years to your life.
- It does this by protecting you from heart disease, hypertension, stroke, diabetes, some forms of cancer, and other chronic diseases.
- Exercise can delay many of the effects of aging, such as bone loss, that can diminish the quality of life among elderly women.
- It is never too late to start a fitness program of any type.

12

Exercise for Women with Chronic Health Conditions

We hope you are convinced by now that moderate physical activity can prevent a variety of illnesses. But can it also do something for people who already have a chronic illness or a serious risk factor for a disease? The answer, in many cases, is a resounding *Yes!*

If you have heart disease, high blood pressure, high cholesterol, diabetes, obesity, osteoporosis, arthritis, or cancer, appropriate physical activity can help you to live a fuller, happier life despite the problem. An activity program can help to ease the symptoms of many medical conditions (or the side effects of treatment), as well as enable you to work with, and even overcome, some of the physical limitations that may result from your illness. In the process, it will improve your mood and help alleviate feelings of depression or doubt that may accompany this change in your physical state.

When 67-year-old Eloise was diagnosed with cervical cancer a week before her 60th birthday, she was surprised, angry, terrified, tearful. "I was devastated. I'd hardly been sick a day in my life before then," said the now-retired postal worker. "I came through surgery OK, but found that the radiation therapy seemed to rob me of my energy." A social worker who specializes in helping people with cancer suggested that Eloise start exercising, even though doing something that might make her even more tired didn't seem to be a very smart solution for relieving fatigue. To her surprise, it worked. "Exercise

215

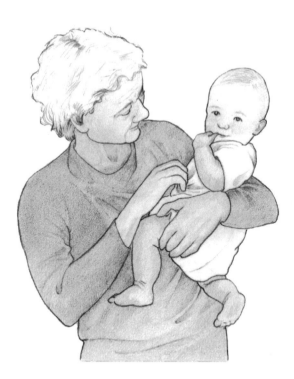

really helped, probably more for psychological reasons than physical ones. Walking through my neighborhood each day, or around the track at the school, made me feel like I was doing something to fight the cancer. I wasn't just having things done to me. Then when the radiation was over, I kept on walking because I figured if it could help me get through something big like that, it sure could help with the smaller stuff."

Moderate activity also helps people cope with a variety of physical ailments. Sarah, the 64-year-old who started doing Volkswalks around the country, uses walking for a variety of problems. "I've been told I have a little arthritis in my knees, and I think walking helps; it keeps the legs moving. I also have high blood pressure, but when my husband takes a blood pressure reading at home after a walk, it seems quite a bit lower. Maybe the walking helps me relax and keeps me cool and calm."

Unfortunately, people with chronic medical conditions are less likely to exercise than people without chronic conditions, even though exercise might benefit them even more. A 1998 study published in the *American Journal of Health Promotion* surveyed 8,000 members of a health maintenance organization who were aged 40 and over. Those with one or more chronic conditions were less physically fit than their healthier counterparts. The researchers concluded that, given the fact that physical activity can actually improve many chronic conditions or at least help people live fuller lives with them, health professionals need to make special efforts to promote physical activity among people living with chronic conditions.

We've gathered exercise recommendations established by major health organizations for people with a variety of medical conditions, so you don't have to start scouring the Internet or a local medical library for them. Please keep in mind that these recommendations— from the American Heart Association, the American Diabetes Association, the American Medical Association, the National Osteoporosis Foundation, the Arthritis Foundation, and others—are very broad. Because everyone is different, *consult your physician before starting any physical activity program—light, moderate, or otherwise—and follow her or his recommendations* (see Box 57).

Exercise and Heart Disease

For many years, prolonged rest was the main therapy for anyone who survived a heart attack, who had undergone bypass surgery, or who had been diagnosed with congestive heart failure or other form of heart disease. That's all changed. Today, moderate exercise is—or should be—an integral and early component of treatment for the millions of people in the United States alone who have survived a heart attack or stroke, undergone angioplasty or bypass surgery, had a heart transplant, or are living with some other form of cardiovascular disease.

Starting an exercise program after having a heart attack or stroke or after finding out that you have some other form of cardiovascular disease may seem like closing the barn door after the horse is gone. It isn't. In fact, there's even more and better proof for the benefits of exercise among people with heart disease than among seemingly healthy people. According to 1995 guidelines drawn up by the federal Agency for Health Care Policy Research, a well-planned cardiac rehabilitation program can help you:

- Feel better faster
- Get stronger
- Reduce stress
- Reduce your chances of having more heart problems in the future
- Live longer

Merely signing up for an exercise program isn't enough—you need to exercise, become more active, and improve your physical fitness. A 20-year follow-up of men who survived a heart attack between 1976 and 1979, for example, showed that those who *enrolled* in an exercise program weren't any less likely to die over the years than those

BOX 57

Workout Tips for Women with Special Medical Problems

- **Check with your doctor:** Whether you are planning a light or moderate workout, always consult your physician before starting any exercise program and follow his or her advice carefully.
- **Warm up:** This helps loosen up stiff muscles and joints, rev up your circulation, and prevent a sudden rise in blood pressure.
- **Avoid high-impact exercises:** These can break blood vessels, harm nerve-damaged feet, injure arthritic joints, and raise blood pressure.
- **Keep warm:** Cold weather stiffens joints and further numbs nerve-damaged feet.
- **Cool down:** After exercising, walk slowly for a few minutes and then stretch. This keeps your joints from stiffening up and also prevents a sudden drop in blood pressure.

who didn't, but the men who actually worked out and became more physically fit over time were less likely to die during the study.

WHAT YOU CAN DO

Cardiac rehabilitation programs must be individually tailored to match your cardiovascular condition, general health, and risk factors for future problems. It's safe to say that if you need such a program, it will have two main thrusts. One is exercise. Expect to start exercising on a treadmill, stationary bicycle, rowing machine, or walking track under the supervision of a clinician. At first, your heart's rate and rhythms, along with your blood pressure, will be closely monitored. You'll be told to start slowly and then urged to gradually increase the duration and intensity of your workouts as you and your heart get stronger.

Not only will the exercise help you return to normal, but you will receive a tremendous amount of emotional support from the physicians, nurses, and exercise physiologists who run the program, as well as from other participants in your supervised program. This psychological support is important because it's not uncommon for patients to feel depressed after a cardiac incident. The combination of exercise and support will show you that you can be healthy and productive again, despite your medical condition. In addition, getting active again may ease concerns that family members have about your health and well-being.

The second part of a cardiac rehabilitation program is an evaluation of your lifestyle and health (or unhealth) habits, with an eye toward finding ways to cut back on, or stop, things that might harm your heart. You will be offered information on how to eat healthier to reduce blood pressure and cholesterol levels. The emphasis here will be on reducing the amount of saturated fats and salt and increasing the amount of fruits, vegetables, and complex carbohydrates in your diet. If you smoke, you'll be offered programs to help you stop smoking. Stress reduction programs are another useful component. They can help you cope with the uncertainty and fears of having heart disease and may also help prevent future heart problems.

Just *having* a cardiac rehabilitation program isn't enough. What's important is that you take charge of your recovery by becoming an active member of the team. For the best results, you also need to view the program as a lifelong venture. Stopping when you feel better may mean a return to the conditions that initially triggered your heart disease.

While the consensus among cardiovascular specialists is that cardiac rehabilitation programs are a key part of treating people with heart disease, less than half of people who could benefit from such programs get them. If you have been diagnosed with, or are recovering from, some form of heart disease and the subject of exercise or cardiac rehabilitation hasn't come up, it's in your best interest to ask about one.

Exercise and High Blood Pressure

High blood pressure, or hypertension, is often called the "silent killer" because it has no symptoms. High blood pressure can damage the arteries in your heart, neck, or brain, and lead to a heart attack or stroke. It is the direct cause of death for more than 40,000 Americans each year and is implicated in another 200,000 deaths a year.

About one in four adults—more than 50 million Americans—have hypertension. In terms of actual blood pressure readings, this means a systolic blood pressure of 140 or higher and/or a diastolic pressure of 90 or higher. A surprising number of people don't know they have high blood pressure. According to the Sixth Report of the Joint National Committee on Prevention, Detection, Evaluation and Treatment of High Blood Pressure (JNC VI), 32% of people with high blood pressure are unaware they have this condition. Of those who do know, 27% are on medication and have their hypertension under control; 26% are on medication but don't have it under control; and 15% are not on medication and don't have it under control.

Who develops high blood pressure? It strikes people of every age, ethnic group, and nationality. It is more common among older people than younger people, though. Only about 6% of men and women under age 35 have high blood pressure. Above this age, the numbers climb steadily—17% of those aged 35 to 44, 30% of those aged 45 to 54, 44% of those aged 55 to 64, 59% of those aged 65 to 74, and a whopping 71% of people over age 75 have high blood pressure.

WHAT YOU CAN DO

If you have high blood pressure, moderate physical activity is one of the first-line therapies that clinicians prescribe, along with losing weight, limiting alcohol intake to a drink a day, reducing the amount of salt and saturated fat in the diet, increasing the amount of calcium and potassium in the diet, and stopping smoking. Depending on how high your blood pressure is, and how resistant it is to lifestyle changes, medication may be added to your prescription.

The JNC VI guidelines, which represent state-of-the-art treatment of hypertension, say this about exercise: "Blood pressure can be lowered with moderately intense physical activity (40 to 60 percent of maximum oxygen consumption), such as 30 to 45 minutes of brisk walking most days of the week." Two warnings: *Avoid really strenuous exertion and high-impact exercise. Both can push blood pressure to a high and possibly dangerous level.* And keep in mind that because this condition has no symptoms, you still need to follow through with whatever therapy has been prescribed for you even when you feel great.

Exercise and High Cholesterol

Until middle age, women tend to have lower cholesterol levels—and thus lower rates of heart disease—than men. But as estrogen levels plummet during and after menopause, women tend to have higher cholesterol levels than men and their rates of heart disease soar. Currently, more than one third of women in the United States age 50 to 59, and more than 40% of those age 60 and older, have high cholesterol, defined as a serum cholesterol level greater than 240 mg/dL.

Getting your cholesterol checked is quick and simple. It doesn't require any special preparation on your part other than sitting for a minute while a nurse or technician draws a tube or two of blood from a vein in your arm. The results, which should be available in a few days, will have two numbers: your total cholesterol level, and the level of a protective form of cholesterol called HDL, which stands for high-density lipoprotein. If the level of total cholesterol is under 200 and HDL is above 35, congratulations—you are in the lucky group with a healthy cholesterol level. If your total cholesterol is over 200 or your HDL is under 35, then your physician may ask you to have what is called a fasting lipid panel to get a more accurate picture of what's in your bloodstream. This time you have to fast for 10 hours before having your blood drawn. The results from this test include not only total cholesterol and HDL but also two other important players—the level of low-density lipoprotein, or LDL (the so-called bad cholesterol), and the level of triglyceride, another type of fatty particle circulating in the blood. Ideally, you hope to see your total cholesterol under 200, your LDL under 160, your HDL over 35, and your triglycerides under 200. If you have too much total cholesterol, LDL, or triglyceride, or too little HDL, your physician will probably recommend some combination of diet and exercise, and possibly drug therapy, depending on (1) how far the levels are from normal, (2) whether or not you have some form of heart disease, and (3) your risk factors for future heart disease.

WHAT YOU CAN DO

The two nondrug approaches to lowering total cholesterol and raising HDL cholesterol are diet and physical activity. Reducing the amount of foods high in cholesterol and saturated fat in the diet can lower levels of total cholesterol and LDL in your bloodstream. Such heart-healthy diets tend to be low in high-fat dairy products and red meat and high in complex carbohydrates, fruits, and vegetables. Your doctor or a dietitian can help you devise a healthy meal plan. In addition, both the American Heart Association and the National Heart, Lung, and Blood Institute have sites on the Internet with tips and recipes for people trying to lower their cholesterol (http://www.deliciousdecisions.org and http://rover.nhlbi.nih.gov/chd/).

Equally important, get moving! In addition to lowering the levels of bad cholesterol, exercise is one of the few ways to increase your level of protective HDL. For these effects, regular moderate exercise such as the regimen recommended by the Surgeon General works just fine.

Exercise, Overweight, and Obesity

Most of us know if we're overweight—we feel it when our clothes stop fitting, or see it when we tug on a bathing suit. But there are health differences between having an extra pound or two and carrying far too many extra pounds. If your weight for height (body-mass index) falls above the healthy zone in the tables in Chapter 5, some action is in order.

WHAT YOU CAN DO

Heed the growing consensus of support for exercising for at least 30 minutes on most days of the week. Strength training twice a week is also important to maintain calorie-burning muscle mass and to build a healthy muscle-to-fat ratio. A National Institutes of Health expert panel on overweight and obesity also recommended increasing everyday activities (http://www.nhlbi.nih.gov/guidelines/obesity/ob_gdlns.htm).

The lower-calorie diet is designed to cause a negative energy balance of 500 to 1,000 calories a day in the energy-in energy- out equation, while the goal of behavior therapy is to help people adjust to and keep up initially uncomfortable and unusual patterns.

Increased physical activity can certainly burn off extra calories each day and may lead to moderate weight loss. All by itself, exercise rarely leads to a dramatic reduction in weight, but it does help you keep off the pounds you've already lost. It also increases resting metabolism, which further helps burn calories. For people who are overweight, the benefits of exercise go far beyond weight loss. Exercise helps increase cells' sensitivity to insulin and thus reduces the risk of developing diabetes. It lowers blood pressure and cholesterol levels, both of which tend to be high in people who are overweight and both of which increase the risk of having a heart attack or developing heart disease.

Exercise and Diabetes

Symptoms of type 2 diabetes tend to develop gradually. These include frequent urination; unusual thirst; extreme hunger; unexplained weight loss; fatigue; blurred vision; irritability; tingling or numbness in the legs, feet, or hands; frequent infections of the skin, gums, vagina, or bladder; itchy skin; and slow healing of cuts and bruises. If you have any of these, see your doctor about being tested for diabetes. If you've already been diagnosed with type 2 diabetes, you may already know that exercise is one of the best things you can do for yourself, along with adopting a healthy diet, managing your weight, and, if needed, taking medication.

WHAT YOU CAN DO

In a recent position statement, the American Diabetes Association said that "it is becoming increasingly clear that exercise may be a therapeutic tool in a variety of patients with, or at risk for, diabetes ... The possible benefits for the patient with type 2 diabetes are substantial, and recent studies strengthen the importance of long-term exercise programs for the treatment and prevention of this common metabolic abnormality and its complications."

While exercise is an important part of controlling diabetes, you need to make sure you are exercising safely and avoiding activities that can make diabetes-related complications worse. The bouncing or pounding that goes along with high-impact aerobics, for example, can aggravate diabetic eye disease or speed up nerve damage. And you have to be prepared for changes in blood sugar that might accompany exercise. Here are some tips for safe, healthy exercise (for both type 1 and type 2 diabetes):

- **Check with your physician before starting an exercise program:** He or she can help you determine the safest before-, during-, and after-exercise blood sugar levels and heart rates, as well as suggest some activities that might be right for you.
- **Buy shoes that fit well:** Protect your feet from blisters and irritation by using silica gel or air insoles that cushion the feet and polyester or cotton-polyester socks that keep them dry.
- **Exercise one to two hours after a meal:** Waiting much longer than that may lead to a precipitous drop in blood sugar. At that pre-exercise meal, drink plenty of fluids, and keep hydrated while exercising, especially on hot days.
- **Test your blood sugar before exercising:** If it is higher than the guidelines set by your physician, wait until the level has fallen into the safe zone. When you have finished exercising, test your blood sugar again.
- **Carry a source of concentrated carbohydrates:** This could be juice,

glucose tablets, or raisins; if your blood sugar level drops, you'll be prepared.

- **Keep hydrated while exercising, especially on hot days.**
- **After exercising, check your feet for blisters or calluses:** This is especially important if you have been diagnosed with the diabetes-related nerve degeneration called peripheral neuropathy.
- **Try not to exercise alone:** And always carry a medical ID or a medical alert bracelet or necklace that mentions you have diabetes.

Two good sources of more detailed information on diabetes and exercise are the booklet *Good Health with Diabetes through Exercise,* available from the Joslin Diabetes Center in Boston (800–344–4501), and *The Fitness Book,* available through the American Diabetes Association (800-DIABETES or http://www.diabetes.org/exercise).

Exercise and Cancer

There was a time when a diagnosis of cancer was a death sentence. While cancer can still be a terrifying and often fatal disease, advances in diagnosis and treatment have allowed more people to survive cancer than die from it. According to the American Cancer Society, more than 8 million Americans alive today are cancer survivors.

Fighting cancer can be a protracted and often draining battle that takes energy, determination, concentration, and support. Sometimes the treatments—radical surgery, radiation therapy, and chemotherapy—seem worse than the disease itself. More and more, cancer experts are recommending that exercise be part of comprehensive treatment and rehabilitation plans.

Why? The National Cancer Institute put it this way: "Exercise (including light- to moderate-intensity walking programs) helps many people with cancer. People with cancer who exercise may have more physical energy, improved ability to function, improved quality of life, improved outlook, improved sense of well being, enhanced sense of commitment, and improved ability to meet the challenges of cancer and cancer treatment. Exercise may also help patients with advanced cancer, even those in hospice care. More benefits may result when family members are involved with the patient in the physical therapy program" (http://www.cancernet.nci.nih.gov/coping/side_effects.shtml).

A number of studies have shown that exercise helps improve energy levels among people who are undergoing chemotherapy or radiation therapy, both of which are notorious for sapping energy. It may reduce pain. It clearly helps maintain muscle strength in the face of treatments that can make muscles atrophy. Studies of women with breast cancer show that exercise improves mood and sleep and reduces depression and anxiety. Cancer survivors also say that exercise is one way to exert some control in a situation where feelings of loss of control can be overwhelming.

WHAT YOU CAN DO

Given the range of cancer types, extents, and treatments, there isn't any one-size-fits-all exercise guideline for people with cancer. Neither the American Cancer Society nor the National Cancer Institute have published any specific recommendations. What we can say, though, is that for some people, exercise is a very useful tool for coping with the emotional shock of a cancer diagnosis, the side effects of treatment, and the uncertainties of life after treatment.

Getting good advice on exercise may not be a simple matter. Your physicians may recommend exercise in general but not be able to recommend a specific program. That's what happened to Jill Forrest, who was diagnosed with breast cancer several years ago. After a modified radical mastectomy, she had difficulty moving her arm. Her doctor suggested she exercise by "walking" her fingers up a wall and clapping her hands over her head, which she just couldn't do. Frustrated by the lack of specifics and worried that the exercises weren't strengthening her muscles, she worked with a certified personal trainer and a plastic surgeon to produce an exercise video specifically for breast cancer survivors. It is called *Better Than Before* and can be ordered by calling 800–488–8354.

Other than creating your own exercise program, you might try contacting the American Cancer Society (800-ACS-2345) or the American Academy of Physical Medicine and Rehabilitation (312–464–9700) for the name of physicians or physical therapists in your area who specialize in cancer recovery.

Exercise and Osteoporosis

Osteoporosis—progressive loss of bone—occurs for a variety of reasons, ranging from not enough calcium in the diet to lack of exercise and use of certain medications. As bones become increasingly fragile, they can break with very little pressure. A misstep off a curb might fracture a bone in the spine, or a fall from a chair onto a carpeted floor might be enough to fracture a hip bone. Hip fractures, which almost always require hospitalization and major surgery, can seriously impair one's ability to walk unassisted and may cause prolonged or permanent disability or death. Spinal or vertebral fractures also have serious consequences, including loss of height, severe back pain, and limited motion.

Ten million Americans (80% of them women) have osteoporosis, and another 18 million are at high risk for developing this condition. Given these numbers, a recent Gallup poll comes as quite a surprise. This survey of women ages 45 to 75 indicates that three out of four women have never spoken to their doctors about osteoporosis. That may be one reason why hip fractures are so common among older women, numbering about 300,000 a year. In fact, a woman's risk of breaking a hip is equal to her combined risk of developing breast, uterine, and ovarian cancer.

WHAT YOU CAN DO

It is never too late to halt this bone-thinning condition. Even if you have already been diagnosed with osteoporosis, you can prevent further bone loss. This usually involves a trio of treatments: increasing the amount of calcium and vitamin D in your diet; taking a medication such as estrogen, calcitonin, alendronate, or raloxifene; and exercise. Calcium and vitamin D are the building blocks of new bone tissue, and medications prime bone cells to build new tissue rather than break down existing bone. Exercise is like the charge that sets the whole bone-building process in motion.

The National Osteoporosis Foundation and the American College of Sports Medicine recommend physical activity as a key part of treating and preventing osteoporosis. There are two direct benefits. Weight-bearing exercise, such as walking, jogging, stair climbing, dancing, and tennis, stimulates bone-building cells and helps maintain bone density, an important factor in resisting breaks. Strength training and stretching exercises improve flexibility, muscle strength, and coordination, all of which prevent loss of balance and falls, which can break fragile bones.

The recently published *Physician's Guide to Prevention and Treatment of Osteoporosis,* developed by the National Osteoporosis Foundation in collaboration with nine medical organizations, says physicians should "recommend regular weight-bearing and muscle-strengthening exercise to reduce the risk of falls and fractures." While the guide doesn't give any specifics, the program we have detailed in this book fills the bill—at least 30 minutes of brisk walking or its equivalent on most days of the week, plus two weekly sessions of strength training and daily stretching exercises.

Your physician may be able to recommend a more specific program for you. Or you might want to check out *Be BoneWise—Exercise,* the official weight-bearing and strength-training exercise video of the National Osteoporosis Foundation. The $19.95 video, which comes with an exercise band and a safe-movement handbook, demonstrates exercises that can be done standing, sitting, and lying down. All of the featured exercises avoid movements that aren't safe for people with osteoporosis, such as twisting the spine or bending forward from the waist. (Available online at http://www.nof.org, or by calling the National Osteoporosis Foundation at 202–223–2226.)

Exercise and Arthritis

"I have arthritis in my knees and in the balls of my feet," explains 66-year-old Maureen. "It's a condition I've had since I was 29. I keep up with my doctor visits because, once in a while, my knees have to be drained of fluid. Five years ago, my son bought a leg extension machine for me. He called my doctor to make sure it was OK, and my doctor said, 'Absolutely yes.' The machine builds up the muscles in the upper part of my leg, so I can move up and down the stairs a lot better. I can feel myself deteriorating when I don't use it, so I do it every day—but only for about five minutes. I do three sets of 10 repetitions using a 1.5 pound weight. Any more is too much for me. I've always been a very active person, and try to walk outside at least five times a week. When I have time, I love to walk on the beach for miles at a stretch. My doctor told me the best thing to do was walk barefoot in the sand in the summer. I feel better when I do it."

Nearly 40 million Americans suffer from arthritis, making it one of the nation's leading causes of disability. The word "arthritis" means joint inflammation, and it actually describes more than 100 specific diseases. Arthritis usually affects the joints as well as the muscles and tendons around them. Some of the most common forms of arthritis include:

- **Osteoarthritis:** a breakdown of joint cartilage, which leads to pain and loss of movement in the joints involved
- **Rheumatoid arthritis:** a disease that turns the immune system against healthy parts of the body, especially the joints
- **Systemic lupus erythematosus:** another autoimmune disease that can damage the skin, kidneys, joints, blood vessels, nervous system, heart, and other internal organs
- **Fibromyalgia:** a painful condition that is accompanied by moderate or severe fatigue, decreased exercise endurance, headaches, and possibly depression

People with arthritis were once told not to exercise because activity would further damage their joints. Today we know that exercise is not only safe but actually helps people with this potentially crippling disease keep their joints moving, the muscles around joints strong, and bones and cartilage strong; and all of these advantages improve their ability to do everyday activities. Not to mention the additional benefits of higher energy levels, better sleep, weight control (which reduces stress on joints), a healthier heart, bones and muscles, and improved mood and attitude.

WHAT YOU CAN DO

The Arthritis Foundation recommends a program that includes three different kinds of exercise: range-of-motion exercises designed to increase flexibility, muscle-strengthening exercises, and endurance exercises. For people with arthritis, the preferred endurance exercises are those that put minimal strain on the joints, such as walking, swimming, or bicycling. Range-of-motion exercises include finger stretches, arm raises, and knee bends. Some strengthening exercises (isometrics) don't involve moving the joints, while others (isotonics) do. *It's important to do strengthening exercises the right way to avoid injuring the joint.* Your physician, physical therapist, or occupational therapist can help design a program that's right for you.

If you are just beginning an exercise program, start out with flexibility and strengthening exercises to loosen your joints and muscles and to get accustomed to exercise. Two or three five-minute sessions a day are a good start. As you feel less stiff and more comfortable, gradually extend the duration of your sessions.

You'll probably need to experiment to find the times of day during which exercise works best for you. Some people prefer exercising in the morning as a way of loosening up for the day ahead; others prefer evening exercise so they don't feel so stiff when they wake up. For each exercise session, the Arthritis Foundation offers these tips:

- Massage stiff or sore areas, or apply heat or cold
- Warm up with easy range-of-motion exercises before walking, swimming, bicycling, or other endurance activity
- Wear comfortable clothes and well-fitting, non-slip, shock-absorbing shoes
- Exercise at a steady pace
- Listen to your body's signals; if exercise is increasing your pain rather than easing it, stop
- Cool down by doing your activity at a slower pace for five to ten minutes—this lets your muscles relax—and try stretching after you've finished

For more information on exercise and arthritis, the Arthritis Foundation publishes a pamphlet called *Exercise and Your Arthritis.* It is available from its Web site (http://www.arthritis.org/answers/exercise_info.asp).

Exercise and Chronic Pain

According to a recent Louis Harris telephone survey, one in five older Americans take painkillers at least several times a week. Previous studies have found that between one quarter and one half of older adults suffer from a fair degree of pain; the proportions are even higher among nursing home residents. Some of the most common causes include low back and shoulder problems, arthritis, osteoporosis, and cancer.

Chronic pain can invade every aspect of one's life, in some cases thoroughly sapping the joy of living. It limits movement and disturbs sleep. It may lead to increased isolation and depression. Constant use of painkillers can cause troubling and potentially serious side effects, as can the interactions among medications. Relatively little is known about the best ways to treat chronic pain. The most common approach has been drug therapy, although a growing body of evidence suggests that exercise and other nondrug therapies can often help reduce pain and, in some cases, eliminate the need for painkilling drugs altogether.

One thing is clear: preventing pain is easier and far more effective than stopping pain once it has started. The nerves that send pain signals to and from the brain aren't just passive relays but are physically changed by pain itself. The more pain signals they receive, the more responsive they become to future pain signals and the more intensely they send "This *hurts*" messages to the brain. Pain isn't good for you—tolerating it doesn't improve your character or make you a stronger, better person. So it's important to do what you can, as soon as you can, to nip pain in the bud.

WHAT YOU CAN DO

Two separate and very different sets of clinical practice guidelines suggest much the same thing—that physical activity and exercise may be important components of any pain-control strategy.

In a recent practice guideline on managing chronic pain in older persons, the American Geriatrics Society says this: "Exercise should be a part of the care of all older patients troubled by chronic pain." Because there is no evidence that one type of exercise is better than another for controlling pain, it is up to you and your physician or physical therapist to establish a plan that appeals to, and works for, you. The society suggests modifying the intensity, frequency, and duration of exercise to avoid making pain worse as you increase and later maintain your overall conditioning. It also cautions that feeling better may give rise to the false hope that the pain is "gone" and that exercise is no longer necessary.

Complex regional pain syndrome (also known as reflex sympathetic dystrophy syndrome) is a puzzling and controversial condition. It starts with an injury—say a broken bone or a severely stubbed toe. Then something goes awry during the healing process, leading to constant, unquenchable pain around the injury that may spread to other parts of the body. (It's controversial because some experts say this is a psychological disorder, while others say it is a physical problem.) New diagnosis and treatment guidelines established by the Reflex Sympathetic Dystrophy Syndrome Association of America encourage the use of physical therapy and exercise to reduce pain and help people with this condition relearn how to use the affected parts of their bodies. Again, the type, intensity, and duration of exercise are left to individuals and their health-care providers.

Exercise and HIV/AIDS

Although the focus of AIDS research has been on finding ways to thwart the virus that causes this gradually debilitating and ultimately fatal disease, one growing branch of research has been concerned with evaluating strategies for living with the disease. Along with drug therapy, exercise and nutrition appear to play key roles.

Regular moderate exercise appears to strengthens the immune system, while overly vigorous activity seems to depress it. A few investigators have applied this knowledge to people who are HIV positive or who have AIDS. Some very small and very preliminary studies suggest that moderate activity may slow the progression of human immunodeficiency virus (HIV) infection. Several small studies have suggested that exercise induces beneficial immune-system changes in people who are HIV positive. A 1999 report appearing in the *Annals of Epidemiology* showed that among a group of 156 HIV-positive men, the progression to full-blown AIDS was slowest among those who exercised three to four times a week and fastest among those who didn't exercise. A few months later, a review in the *New England Journal of Medicine* pointed to exercise as a "potentially promising strategy," either alone or in combination with appetite-boosting drugs, for a condition called AIDS wasting. This syndrome, one of the conditions that defines the change from being HIV positive to having AIDS, is a gradual, involuntary loss of weight, often accompanied by diarrhea, weakness, and fever.

Until fairly recently, heart disease and other aging- or lifestyle-related conditions just weren't an important issue for people infected with HIV. But thanks to a number of new drugs that have been developed to suppress the activity and replication of HIV, people who are HIV positive are living longer and longer. As with all drugs, these have unwanted side effects. For example, the type of drug therapy responsible for this increased survival, known as highly active antiretroviral therapy, can lead to a redistribution of body fat around the trunk and abdomen, the pattern most associated with increased risk of diabetes and heart disease. A pilot study from Tufts University School of Medicine showed that a combination of strength training and aerobic exercise can reduce abdominal fat in men who have this drug-related redistribution, which goes by the name lipodystrophy.

It is too early to tell if exercise will, indeed, slow the progression of HIV infection or AIDS wasting. But all the benefits of exercise that apply to a general population also apply to people with HIV. Exercise builds a stronger, more efficient heart and lungs, improves muscle strength and flexibility, helps the body handle blood sugar more efficiently, decreases stress, improves mood and body image, and may generate a sense of mastery.

WHAT YOU CAN DO

So far, no specific guidelines have been established for the role of exercise in treating, or coping with, HIV infection or AIDS. That means you will need to talk through different options with your physicians and other health-care providers. Different strategies will be appropriate for different people, or at different stages of infection.

- If you have no symptoms of HIV infection and are otherwise healthy, the regimen we have been suggesting throughout this book should work for you—moderate exercise lasting 30 minutes or more 3 to 5 times a week, supplemented with two weekly sessions of strength training and daily stretching. Approach extremely vigorous activities, such as training for a marathon, with some caution and consult your health-care provider, because this kind of activity has been shown to weaken immune system activity. Make sure that you are eating enough to take care of your body's needs as well as the extra calories you're burning off.

- If you are symptomatic, or are recovering from an HIV-related illness, how much you exercise should be dictated by how well you feel, measures of your immune system activity, and guidance from your physicians. If you are just starting an exercise program, start with gentle exercises and slowly build your endurance. If you are returning to an exercise program, the same thing holds true—don't try to jump in where you left off.

Exercise and Physical or Mental Disabilities

"Individuals with disabilities, for the most part, can gain very similar benefits from physical activity and the accrued physical fitness as people without disabilities." That's the conclusion of a report on physical activity for people with disabilities from the President's Council on Physical Fitness and Sports.

WHAT YOU CAN DO
As in several other cases, there are no official guidelines to help plan or direct exercise programs for people with disabilities. Here again, the Surgeon General's recommendation of at least 30 minutes of moderate activity on most days of the week plus two strength-training sessions a week is a good starting place.

- Target heart rate isn't always the best way to measure the intensity of exercise for people with disabilities. People with Down syndrome, for example, may not be able to reach their target because of possible heart-valve damage. People with quadriplegia usually can't sustain heart rates much higher than 120 beats per minute. And fatigue may keep people with multiple sclerosis from reaching their targets. Sometimes the *perception* of exertion is just as important as hitting an actual target.
- Strength training should be done carefully and with a "spotter," especially if a disability causes poor posture, limited range of motion, or problems with balance or stability. Resistance or weight

machines tend to be safer because they allow only a limited path of motion. Free weights offer greater exercise options, since they come in a variety of sizes, but require more balance and coordination. A carefully designed strength-training program may benefit people with muscular dystrophy, multiple sclerosis, polio, or other conditions that cause a slow degeneration of muscle, but it shouldn't be started without consulting a physician.

Where to Find Help

If you have a chronic condition, by all means check with your doctor about appropriate exercise. Then you might want to contact your local YMCA/YWCA, Jewish Community Center (JCC), hospital wellness center, or private health club for an exercise program that is suited to your special needs. Check your Yellow Pages to find a YMCA/YWCA or a Jewish Community Center. You can call the Y's national headquarters at 800–872–9622, or find it on the World Wide Web at http://www.ymca.net/; the telephone number for the JCC's national headquarters is 212–532–4949, and its Web site is http://www.jcca.org.

To find a private health club with appropriate programming, visit www.healthclubs.com, and use the search engine to find a club near you. This is the commercial site for the International Health, Racquet and Sportsclub Association (IHRSA), an organization of nearly 3,000 for-profit U.S. clubs. According to the latest report, 69 percent of IHRSA clubs had a weight-loss program, 65 percent had wellness education, 62 percent had senior fitness, 61 percent had aquatics programs, 33 percent had physical therapy, and 32 percent had cardiac rehabilitation programs. Nearly 30 percent of these clubs are affiliated with hospitals. At some clubs you must be a member to take advantage of their programs, while others make these programs available to nonmembers as well. For guidelines for finding a high-quality health club that suits your needs, see Box 47.

Points to Remember

- If you have a chronic medical condition, such as heart disease, high blood pressure, high cholesterol, overweight or obesity, diabetes, cancer, arthritis, or osteoporosis, exercise can ease the symptoms associated with the condition, possibly improve the condition itself, and improve your mental outlook.

- Your doctor should be your primary resource and contact about exercise. Guidelines from a number of major medical organizations can also help direct your exercise program.

- Don't overlook the exercise opportunities available at many YMCA/YWCAs, JCCs, hospital wellness centers, or private health clubs.

13

Working the Body, Healing the Mind

Ask anyone who exercises regularly why she does it and she will probably tell you it's a survival tactic that's essential for coping with life's challenges. Chances are she will describe her exercise sessions as something so important to her mental health and well-being that it's difficult to think of a day without it. Maybe she'll acknowledge that it's sometimes tough to get started on any given day, but once she gets going exercise makes her feel much better. Or she might tell you that problems which seem insurmountable before a workout can feel manageable, even inconsequential, afterward. How exercise has become a priority for her. How she makes time. How important it is to her mood and outlook. How she feels before and after.

So powerful are the effects of exercise and physical activity on the mind that they have been found to be important aids for people who are trying to quit their addiction to drugs, cigarettes, and alcohol. Physical activity is also increasingly used as one part of multifaceted approaches to treating depression, anxiety, and other psychological and emotional problems. Indeed, both the short-term and long-term mental and emotional benefits of exercise have been well documented. As the 1996 Surgeon General's report on *Physical Activity and Health* states, regular physical activity may:

- Improve your mood
- Reduce anxiety

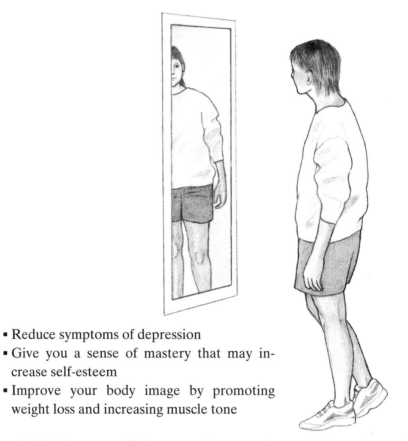

- Reduce symptoms of depression
- Give you a sense of mastery that may increase self-esteem
- Improve your body image by promoting weight loss and increasing muscle tone

In this chapter, we'll document the research on exercise and mood and talk about one other issue that affects many women—body image. A positive body image is an essential component of mental health, and research clearly shows that even a small amount of moderate exercise can improve the way you feel about your body.

Improvements in "State" and "Trait"

The connection between physical activity and mental health dates back thousands of years. In ancient China, physical activity was seen as an integral component of health and "harmony with the world." In India, prescriptions for physical activity in use as early as 3000 BC eventually developed into yoga, a philosophy based on the integration of mind and body. Hippocrates and Galen, the Greek physicians whose writings formed the foundation of early medicine, often described the connection between physical activity and mental health.

Interest in this topic has captured the attention of modern scientists and physicians as well. Hundreds of large and small studies have examined many different aspects of the connection between physical activity and mental health. Because studying people is a tricky task, and because there are so many different variables involved, we can't say there's rock-solid, indisputable proof that exercise brings about improvement in all forms and types of depression in all people, or that it makes everyone happier. There is, however, more than enough evidence to recommend the use of exercise as one method of battling the blues, unknotting tension, or calming anxiety. It can also help you feel better about yourself.

Researchers have used a variety of benchmarks in looking at physical activity and mental health. So-called *state* measures reflect how someone feels "right now." They are often used to look at changes in mood that may occur with a single bout of activity. So-called *trait* measures reflect more stable personality characteristics. They are used to assess how someone "generally" feels and so can help detect changes wrought by physical activity over the long term. Another way scientists have approached this issue is to look at large samples of people and to compare the rates of depression, anxiety, or other psychological or emotional problems among those who are most active and those who are least active.

The consensus from such studies indicates that exercise:

- **Can act as an antidepressant:** People with symptoms of depression, as well as those diagnosed with clinical depression, benefit from increased physical activity and exercise. Even single sessions of exercise lead to reductions in symptoms of depression. Apparently, the antidepressant effects of exercise appear right away and may persist for a while after a person stops his or her exercise program. There also seems to be a dose-response relationship when it comes to depression—the more one exercises, within reason, the greater the antidepressant effect.
- **Can reduce anxiety:** All by itself, exercise can make an anxious person less anxious. Depending on the study, activity-induced reduc-

tions ranged from small to moderate and occurred in all types of people regardless of the intensity or duration of the exercise or whether or not the exercise was done consistently (so-called chronic exercise) or in occasional spurts (acute exercise). This research supports something you may have already discovered on your own—if you are anxious over, say, an upcoming business meeting, deadline, or appointment with your doctor, exercise can help dissipate some of the tension.

- **Can enhance self-esteem and mood:** Exercise significantly increases self-esteem and improves mood. Even in studies that showed no overall physical changes in response to exercise, participants often reported feeling physically, psychologically, or socially better off after exercise.

- **Can improve sleep:** Both strength training and aerobic exercise have been shown to increase the deep phase of sleep known as slow-wave sleep (which is more restful than rapid eye movement or REM sleep), increase total sleep time, and decrease the time it takes to fall asleep and the amount of time spent in REM sleep. It can improve sleep for "normal sleepers" as well as for people routinely plagued by problems getting to sleep or staying asleep. This holds true for older people, who are more prone to insomnia or interrupted sleep than younger people. Exercise which takes place earlier in the day rather than later appears to have the greatest effect on sleep.

As a Coping Mechanism

How does physical activity work this mental magic? Researchers believe that exercise increases the concentrations of at least two chemical messengers in the brain, dopamine and serotonin, both of which are related to mood. Exercise also increases the levels of natural opiates called endorphins and enkephalins that act like painkillers and also enhance mood. These chemical changes last two to four hours after an exercise session.

For some people, the positive physical and mental changes induced by exercise feel so good that they experience a kind of withdrawal when they skip an exercise session. Of course, this is not an addiction in the real sense (except in the case of extreme amounts of activity). Once exercise becomes a habit, most people simply begin to *rely* on the mood-altering and stress-reduction benefits.

Joan, who has battled depression for many of her 38 years, has learned to use exercise as a tool to improve her moods and to cope with the sometimes difficult transitions that have occurred in her adult life. Here she describes how exercise helped her relieve the extreme stress caused by an unexpected job loss, a move to another city, and job-hunting in her new location.

"When my law firm opened a New York office in 1991, I moved there from Boston. It was a stressful move, so I decided to find a new gym right away. I followed the same exercise routine I had done in Boston. I gained strength, I had more energy, and slept better because I was less stressed. But then I was laid off. I continued to work out—if I had nothing to do on a particular day but write letters to employers about jobs, exercise gave a focus and structure to the day. Exercise was a chance to get out of my apartment and do something constructive. I had control over it; I could see results. I could improve one area of my life, and feel masterful."

Exercise and "Girl Power"

If you usually complete your daily walking sessions alone or with a partner, we also encourage you to participate in the fitness walks or fun runs that may be held in your community. While a solitary walk has its benefits, fitness events involving large groups of people provide an oft-needed social venue, in addition to being just plain fun. Such events celebrate health, fitness, confidence, and mastery, and encourage feelings of community and belonging. Many also benefit a worthy cause—an added plus for participants. All of these things enhance mental health and emotional well-being.

One example is the Tufts Health Plan 10K for Women, a road race held every Columbus Day in Boston. At the 23rd annual running of this race, nearly 6,500 women of all sizes, shapes, ages, and fitness levels participated. Helicopters buzzed overhead, police rerouted traffic, volunteers handed out cups of water, and 20,000 friends, family, and city residents cheered the women on.

One onlooker standing on an overpass flashed a sign reading "Girl Power," while a hard-hitting Madonna song blared from a boom box. The sign and the song made some women cheer and raise their arms in victory. The race course, which begins atop historic Beacon Hill on Boston Common, continues downhill to quaint Charles Street, then over the Charles River into Cambridge, where it passes in front of the Massachusetts Institute of Technology. It crosses over the river again to Boston's Back Bay, then finishes where it started, at Boston Common, where free food and refreshments await the runners.

"This was my first Tufts 10K and I'm so glad that I decided to do it," says 30-year-old Barb. "Hearing the cheering crowds along the race route, and seeing women of all ages and fitness levels supporting each other while achieving the same goal was very exciting. Completing the race was an extremely empowering experience for me."

Races like the Tufts 10K are all about girl power—not just for the winning runner, a world-class athlete, but for every woman who makes the effort, who puts on her jogging shoes and completes her workouts on days when she feels like it and days when she doesn't. It doesn't matter if she finishes the course in 30 minutes or three hours—each woman is there to run the best she can. In doing so, she is a celebrity for a day to her partner, her children, her friends, and herself.

Mona, a Tufts participant who is now in her 70s, enjoys a very active retirement. She is motivated by her own pleasant memories of an active childhood in the country and by her mother's good example to create an active, healthy lifestyle—one that has only improved with age. It was not until her 50s, however, that Mona discovered that running in women's races and hiking in beautiful locations around the world could add an extra measure of richness and satisfaction to her life.

"When I started, I was appalled; I could run only half a block. But I built up quite quickly—to five miles. I don't know when I ran my first road race; it was by accident. I went with a friend to what we thought was a fun run, but it was a race. I began to do the women's road races on Mother's Day, and I've done one every year since except for the year I took at trip to the U.K. to climb its highest mountain. I run 10K races now, and I've taken second or third in my age division several times. This year in the Tufts race I took second place in my division—though you don't have to point out that there aren't many women in their 70s running 10K races. It's a great satisfaction. The spirit among the women is wonderful. I don't know when I would ever want to stop."

Body Image: A Watershed Issue for Many Women

When it comes to emotional well-being, few would disagree that many women are troubled by their body image. Consider the following scene. Has this, or a variation, happened to you or a friend?

It is a sunny, Sunday afternoon at Tanglewood, the summer home of the Boston Symphony Orchestra in Lenox, Massachusetts. Five women of various ages sit in a circle on the grass, eating picnic lunches. The orchestra shed stands in front of the group, the stage set for the day's performance. Behind the women, the green, rolling hills of the Berkshires are shrouded in hazy heat.

The friendly chatter among the group, strangers who have met for the first time on a chartered bus, centers at first around heavy traffic encountered during the 150-mile trip from the city, the day's good weather, and the afternoon's musical offerings. However, it isn't long before the subject turns to the food in front of them, and to weight problems and body fat. The tone of the talk becomes decidedly guilt-ridden and self-critical.

One of the women, a physician in her late 30s, speaks with a surprising harshness about her body as she nibbles at a light snack. Her weight appears to be perfectly appropriate for her height; the muscle tone in her upper body suggests that she strength trains on a regular basis, and, in fact, she speaks of regular trips to the gym. Yet she complains with an air of sad resignation that her pear-shaped body carries most of its bulk in her hips and thighs.

If anything about this scene sounds familiar, that's not surprising. For many women, the mere mention of food, exercise, or some related issue will often elicit groans of dissatisfaction. As a 1997 *Psychology Today* survey on body image pointed out, while we have grown heavier over the years, our body preferences have grown thinner. In the 1950s, the epitome of womanhood, Marilyn Monroe, was 5'5" and 135 pounds. That's a far cry from the tall, willowy models we see today on the runways of New York and Paris.

Psychology Today's survey revealed that most women aren't happy with two related conditions—how much they weigh and how they look. Overall, 89% of the 3,500 women who responded to the survey said they wanted to lose weight, and 56% said they weren't satisfied with their appearance. Specifically, 71% were unhappy with their abdomens, 60% disliked their hips, and 58% did not like their muscle tone. An astounding one quarter of the respondents said they would give up more than three years of their lives to achieve their ideal weight! Such feelings were as common among the older women who took part in the survey as they were among the younger women.

Improving Body Image Takes Time

If you have had a negative body image most of your life, you can change it, over time, with consistent effort. Consider the experience of 26-year-old Helen, who despite being overweight as a child and gaining and losing between 10 and 65 pounds several times throughout her life, is gradually learning to put the emphasis where it belongs—on health more than on appearance. Still, improving her body image is something she continues to work on.

"Growing up, I had a brother who tortured me for being overweight. I'd seen my mother, who was beautiful when she was young, put on weight. When I feel out of control, I don't exercise at all, and I eat everything in sight. When I feel bad about myself, and I see some thin girl eat something fattening, I'll catch myself thinking that it's not fair that she can eat that food and I can't. While I did lose 65 pounds, it has been a struggle the last few months. I'd have a good month, then I'd start staring at my imperfections in the mirror. It's so amazing how my mindset can change so drastically. I thought that my life would come together magically when I lost weight, but that didn't happen. I had unrealistic expectations about how it was going to change my life. My self worth is so tied to the way I look. The weight is an emotional cushion against the world."

"At the same time, I've gained a new respect for myself from the weight loss. I don't know how I did it. I may be up 15 pounds right now, but I'm OK. I'm looking forward to a new start tomorrow. I know that preserving muscle mass is more important than a decrease on the scale. Instead, I pay attention to what the tape measure says.

The weight loss will occur over time. I know that my good lifestyle practices will pay off down the road."

Exercise to Improve Your Body Image

If you have a problem with your body image, the combination of regular exercise, strength training, and a sensible diet can help your body become more toned over a 6- to 12-month period. Equally important, that same amount of exercise can help you *feel better about the way you look* and maybe even to appreciate your body for the marvel that it is.

In the *Psychology Today* survey, respondents reported that exercise generated positive feelings about body image and that even moderate exercise did the trick. Similar results have been reported from studies with even greater scientific rigor. For example, in a 1998 study at the Chattanooga Lifestyle Center in Tennessee, 75 women whose average weight was 193 pounds completed two 15-minute sessions of light cardiovascular activity per week. At the beginning of the study, the women were tested in several mood categories including tension/anxiety, depression/dejection, and fatigue. When they took the same tests just two months later, their scores showed dramatic improvements in these categories. Not only that, their vigor jumped significantly and there was a corresponding improvement in how the women felt about themselves. Tests also showed substantial increases in satisfaction with overall appearance and improved perceptions of fitness and health. Not only were these positive feelings good in themselves but they also encouraged the women to keep exercising.

"These dramatic changes occurred despite the fact that circumference measures and actual weight changed very little," says James Annesi, who orchestrated the study. "On a one-to-ten scale, while the actual changes were well under a 1, the perceptual changes were a 10. Because these positive changes continued throughout the 12 weeks of the study (and were emphasized with participants), the adherence rate for these women was very high. In other words, these positive feelings helped these women form the beginning of an exercise habit."

There's a critical take-home message from this research. As you exercise, do it for one reason—your health—and let changes in your physiology be an attractive by-product of your improved health. While it is true that many people do exercise to control weight, any weight loss from regular moderate exercise is likely to occur over a long period of time, often at least 6 months.

So for the first 6 months of your exercise program, try to focus on metabolic changes such as a lower resting heart rate as reinforcement that you are, indeed, making progress. As regular exercise becomes a necessary part of your daily routine, you'll feel better about the way you look, and gain a greater sense of control over your life. Eventually, if you are supplementing your exercise program with a moderate diet, you will see some weight loss.

If you include strength training in your program, you may experience a small and temporary weight gain even as your clothes begin to fit more loosely, simply because you will be adding a small amount of muscle, and muscle weighs more than fat. However, improving your muscle-to-fat ratio will boost your metabolism (and thus boost your weight-loss efforts), protect you from injury, tone your body, and build your self-esteem and confidence. If you haven't started to strength train at this point, we urge you to refer to Chapter 8 and get started right away.

Here are some other important tips for further improving your body image:

- **Focus your attention elsewhere:** Mood is clearly linked to self-image. The days when nothing seems to go right are the days when we are most critical of how we look, the days when even a favorite piece of clothing looks awful. At these times in life, it's best to distract yourself. Better yet, give yourself something else you can be proud of. Get out and take a brisk walk—odds are it will improve your mood. If you've wanted to take a class in painting or piano, get on the phone and sign up for one. If you've been meaning to call a friend or relative, do it. If you've intended to file those stacks of papers at work or clean out the basement, get started. The point is to give your self a sense of pride about who you are and what you can do, rather than focus on how you look. Once you feel better about yourself mentally, you'll feel more comfortable with your physical self.

- **Reward yourself:** If you are like most American women, you constantly juggle work and family. One way to feel better about yourself is to take time off whenever you can and give yourself a treat. If you can afford it, go have a massage or pedicure, or change your hair color or cut. When you have time, take a leisurely hot bath with a special soap or bath oil. Get out the blender and make yourself a fruit smoothie, and then sip it slowly. In the summer, buy a new plant for your perennial garden or cut flowers for the living room. In the winter, pick out a warm, soft pair of wool socks and pay a few extra dollars for cashmere. Giving yourself some sensual pleasures will help you feel good inside and out.
- **Use positive self-talk:** Barring negative comments from someone else, how you feel is determined largely by your own internal dialogue. If you look in the mirror and allow yourself to think "my thighs are ugly" or "my stomach is too fat," you will continue to feel bad about yourself. If, however, you continue to give yourself positive messages—"my legs are really strong" or "this body has borne three wonderful children" or "I'm really working at being my best"—you will begin to feel better. Try to show yourself the same kindness and compassion that you would afford to others.

Points to Remember

- Exercise can improve your mood, reduce anxiety, reduce symptoms of depression, enhance your self-esteem, improve your body image, and help you to sleep better.
- Researchers believe these changes come about through alterations in brain chemistry and increases in body temperature, which improve your mood and relax you.
- Large-group fitness activities also inspire feelings of community and camaraderie.
- Exercise can also promote a healthy body image—a major issue for many women.

14

Fitness at Each Stage
of Your Life

Like compound interest, the benefits of exercise accrue over time.
The solid foundations you establish early in life will help you maintain a healthy, active life. But even if you don't start until middle age
or later, regular physical activity can still contribute to a healthier old
age. In fact, there is a tremendous amount of scientific evidence indicating that it is never too late to reap some benefit from becoming
more active.

Your body has already seen remarkable changes, and more are
surely to come. You've grown from a tiny, helpless babe that your
mother could cradle in the crook of her arm to a woman who could
do such cradling herself. Along the way you grew up and out,
sprouted breasts, started menstruating. Your teen years dragged by
as your body made the sometimes tough transition from girl to
woman. As an adult, you may have gone through the truly astounding changes that accompany pregnancy and childbirth. Or perhaps
you've been watching fine wrinkles appear around your eyes and
mouth, sensing parts of your body sag a bit, or feeling that your muscles aren't as strong as they used to be. The changes in your outlook,
your responsibilities, and your relationships have probably been just
as astounding. At every stage of your biological and emotional development, regular, moderate exercise can help you stay healthy, cope
with stress, and ease you through the many transitions of a full life.

In this chapter, we will describe the benefits of regular physical ac-

248

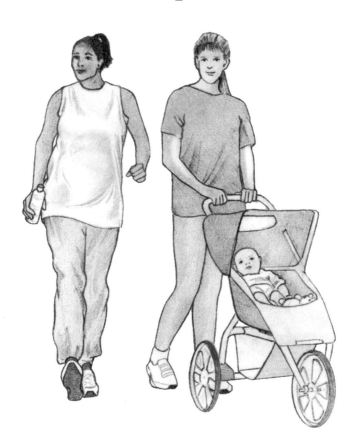

tivity during the key stages of a woman's life and offer some simple recommendations.

Exercise for Teens and Young Women

During the early stage of a woman's life, exercise can accomplish many things. Some of its benefits are:

- Helping form a life-long exercise habit
- Reaching peak bone mass
- Building confidence and self-esteem
- Coping with premenstrual symptoms
- Maintaining a healthy prepregnancy weight

RECOMMENDATION

Girls in their teens and young adult women in their 20s should, at a minimum, engage in 30 minutes of moderate, weight-bearing exercise each day, such as walking or an aerobics class. In addition, they should incorporate two to three sessions of strength-training exercises per week which make use of the major muscle groups of the body (see Chapter 8). To avoid injury, it is important to allow a resting period of 48 to 72 hours between strength-training workouts.

Starting a daily exercise routine early in life, rather than later, has a number of advantages. First, because girls tend to reach their peak bone mass by age 20, strength training during the teen years can ensure that bones reach their full potential in terms of strength and density. Second, starting an exercise habit before age 20 may simply be easier than at age 40 or 50. As you get older, it can become more difficult—though it certainly is possible—to establish new routines. Third, regular activity begun early in life helps keep off much of the weight that many women tend to gain as they age.

For many young women, participation in high school and college sports can be a great way to make friends, build confidence, encourage self-discipline, and establish the beginning of a lifelong exercise habit. If, for example, you run track, play tennis, or join your school soccer team, the odds are high that you will stay interested in running or tennis or soccer for the rest of your life. Even if you stop these sports for a long period, you will probably be able to pick them up again later because they are familiar, because you have a natural affinity for them, because participation gives you feelings of mastery and confidence, and because you remember they were fun.

At the same time, when it comes to participation in competitive sports—or any prolonged, vigorous exercise training, for that matter—some caution is in order. Frequent, prolonged vigorous training (five or more sessions per week lasting 90 minutes or longer would be considered excessive for most people) may cause irregular menstrual periods due to a drop in body fat and body weight. Sometimes periods stop altogether. This condition, called amenorrhea, can definitely affect a woman's ability to become pregnant. It can also lead to bone thinning and fractures.

Some women who exercise to excess may be suffering from a syndrome known as the female athlete triad. First recognized in female athletes, this serious problem affects many women in our society who feel tremendous pressure to be thin. That pressure may lead to disordered eating habits such as self-starvation (anorexia nervosa) or binge eating followed by vomiting or laxatives (bulimia nervosa). These serious problems can be connected to excessive exercise, which is often a substitute for vomiting or laxatives. The third component of the triad, amenorrhea and subsequent osteoporosis, is an end result of the first two behaviors.

The female athlete triad can lead to serious problems. Anorexia nervosa and bulimia nervosa can damage the heart and digestive system; the death rate among women with these eating disorders may be as high as 18%. Also, instead of helping to build up peak bone mass for a lifetime of strong, healthy bones, this condition may lead to early osteoporosis. Some young women with exercise-induced amenorrhea have the reduced bone mass of 70-year-old women!

Those risks aside, we can't emphasize enough how important it is for young women to engage in regular, moderate-to-vigorous activity. It can reduce stress, improve your mental outlook, and even relieve some of the symptoms associated with premenstrual syndrome. In addition, if you plan to have a child at some time in the future, you'd be smart to start your exercise routine and healthy eating habits now to maintain a healthy weight. A 1998 study published in the *New England Journal of Medicine,* for example, showed that overweight women were three times more likely to have a late miscarriage, and obese women four times more likely, than leaner women. Overweight women were also more likely to deliver their first babies prematurely.

Exercise for Pregnant Women

For many women, pregnancy is a time of settling in, of planning and preparing, of sudden bouts of exhaustion and mood swings and dramatic body changes. Exercise can help in many ways:

- By providing more energy and decreasing fatigue
- By improving muscle tone and endurance

- By preventing excess weight gain
- By improving digestion and reducing constipation
- By improving posture and reducing the back pain often associated with pregnancy
- By easing the symptoms of stress, anxiety, and depression that may be associated with pregnancy

RECOMMENDATION

Guidelines from the American College of Obstetricians and Gynecologists (ACOG) state clearly that most women can exercise throughout pregnancy, within limits, if they take certain precautions. Moderate exercise three to five times a week is better than intermittent exercise. Avoid any type of exercise that could lead to abdominal injury. Make sure you don't get overheated. And make sure you get enough fluids and are eating well.

As soon as you discover that you are pregnant, be sure to ask about physical activity during your pregnancy the first time you see your doctor or midwife. Generally speaking, pregnancy is not the best time to start a new regimen of vigorous activity. It is a perfectly fine time, though, to start a walking program, provided that you start gradually, paying close attention to how you feel.

Because exercise during and after pregnancy has many benefits, many health clubs, YMCAs, and park and recreation districts now offer prenatal and postnatal exercise classes which encourage healthy activity at the appropriate level of intensity.

If you were active before you became pregnant—if you swam, jogged, played tennis, danced, or walked regularly—there is a very good chance that you can continue these activities as long as you keep your heart rate under 140 beats per minute. If you can carry on a conversation while you exercise, your heart rate is probably below 140. Don't be surprised if you can't do the same things you did before you got pregnant, or notice a decline in your athletic "performance." In a study of runners, aerobic dancers, and cross-country skiers, 60% said they noticed a substantial drop in their exercise performance during pregnancy.

How safe is vigorous exercise for pregnant women, and what effects does it have? One recent study from the Columbia School of Public Health showed that vigorous exercise does not raise the risk of pre-term delivery and may actually lead to more timely deliveries. In a study of 557 middle-class pregnant women, the well-conditioned exercisers tended to deliver at full term, and their deliveries were faster than those of the nonexercisers.

Because every woman, and every pregnancy, is different, your doctor or midwife is in the best position to help you determine a safe and healthy level of activity. Her or his recommendations will probably reflect the American College of Obstetricians and Gynecologists' recommendations summarized below and in Box 58:

- If you were doing weight-bearing exercise before pregnancy, you will probably be able to continue after consulting with your clinician. However, consider non-weight-bearing exercises such as swimming or cycling, which are less likely to cause injury during pregnancy. Regular exercise is better than an on-again, off-again approach.
- Vigorous exercise draws blood away from the uterus to the limbs, so mild to moderate exercise is generally safer for your baby than vigorous exercise.
- Because the uterus presses down on veins that return blood to the heart, after the first trimester avoid standing still in one position for long stretches, as you might do with some kinds of weight lifting. If you lift weights, try to move and reposition your lower body whenever possible. Also, avoid exercises that require you to lie on your back (known as the supine position), as this position also reduces blood flow.
- During pregnancy, your body needs more oxygen even when you are sitting still or sleeping than it did before your pregnancy. That means you might get winded or tire more easily with exercise. Closely monitor the way you feel during exercise and modify the intensity of your workouts accordingly. If you begin to feel tired, stop exercising and by all means don't exercise to exhaustion. When you exercise, dress appropriately and drink enough fluids so that your body does not overheat.
- Avoid any type of exercise that leads to a loss of balance, especially in the third trimester, because a fall may cause harm to you or to your baby. Also avoid activities that might lead to even mild blows to the abdomen.

BOX 58

When to Avoid Exercise during Pregnancy

DO NOT exercise if you have any of the following conditions:

- Pregnancy-induced hypertension
- Preterm rupture of the membranes
- Preterm labor (or if you experienced it during a prior pregnancy)
- Incompetent cervix
- Persistent second-to-third trimester bleeding
- Slowing of the baby's growth

STOP exercising and consult you physician immediately if you develop any unusual symptoms, such as:

- Discharges from the vagina
- Sudden swelling in the ankles
- Swelling, pain, or redness in one calf, hands, or face
- Severe, persistent headaches
- Fainting or dizzy spells
- Excessive fatigue
- Palpitations or chest pain
- Unexplained abdominal pain
- Weight loss or insufficient weight gain
- Persistent contractions that may signal premature labor

- Pregnancy requires an additional 300 calories per day. If you exercise, make sure that your diet provides the additional calories required by both your pregnancy and your physical activity.

Exercise Following Pregnancy

Now that your baby is here, you probably want your "old body" back. For a few lucky women, that happens all by itself. For most, though, it takes some effort. Physical activity is a critical element in this process. It can help:

- Restore muscle strength and flexibility
- Minimize fatigue
- Return the body to its pre-pregnancy weight and shape
- Maintain a positive outlook

RECOMMENDATION

Many of the physiological changes that accompany pregnancy last for one to two months after delivery. During this postpartum period, it makes good sense to follow the guidelines that apply to exercise during pregnancy. Most new mothers find their strength and flexibility diminished after delivery. Several exercises can help. Kegel exercises can help restore vaginal tone. When you feel that your body is ready to handle a bit more exercise, start a gradual, brisk walking program. One good way to do this is through a postnatal exercise program at a local health club, YMCA, or recreation department. If you had a cesarean section or any other complication during pregnancy or delivery, your doctor or midwife will advise you when it's OK to begin an exercise program.

Regular exercise can help to return your body to its prepregnancy weight and shape. And though it sounds contradictory, exercise can also help reduce the fatigue that many new mothers experience. Equally important, it may also combat one of the most startling "complications" of motherhood. Although the arrival of a new baby is usually a happily anticipated event, many new moms get the "maternity blues." No one knows exactly what causes depression after delivery. The culprit(s) may include abrupt hormonal changes, the stress of caring for a baby (especially one who won't nurse or has colic), lack of help and support, or the sudden change in your relationship with your partner. Exercise is an excellent way to help work off these blues. The signs of the maternity blues—tiredness, anxiety, irritability, and mood swings—resemble those of depression. If they persist, or start to worry you, check with your clinician.

Exercise for Women Ages 40 to 55

Though middle age has never been accorded the glamour and excitement associated with other phases of life, it's a very important and often extraordinarily busy time. Biologically, it is also a very important time for exercise. Continuing a pattern of physical activity established early in life, or starting one now, can help:

- Maintain muscle mass
- Keep bones strong
- Lose weight that may have been gained during pregnancy or as a result of middle-aged spread
- Maintain joint strength and flexibility
- Maintain a positive outlook

RECOMMENDATION

The Surgeon General's recommendations on physical activity apply squarely to this group of women—30 minutes of moderate to vigorous activity every day, if possible, plus two sessions of strength training per week.

One of the most common complaints of women in their 40s is the malady called middle-aged spread. By age 45, most of us are carrying around at least eight pounds of fat we didn't have in our 20s. And the hormonal changes that accompany menopause threaten to add more. In addition, this is a time when bone loss begins in earnest, and muscles begin to lose their flexibility and strength.

For these reasons, it is essential for middle-aged women who hope to live long, healthy lives to engage in regular aerobic exercise and strength training. Regular activity preserves bone mass and strength, which is important throughout a woman's lifetime. Exercise can help us cope with the stress and mood changes that may occur in midlife— as our kids leave home, as we take on more challenging jobs in the workplace or rejoin the workforce after years of raising children, or as we face caring for aging parents or ill partners or divorce. In short, exercise can help you maintain a feeling of control at a time of many important and often stressful transitions.

Menopause is certainly one of the major transitions that women face during this life stage, and it triggers a range of emotional and psychological responses. It also triggers a number of physiological responses, some of which can make life both unpredictable and downright uncomfortable. These include hot flashes, sleeping problems, fatigue, mood swings, and depression. Exercise can help keep these under control.

Three of four women experience hot flashes during menopause, and up to 10 percent are still getting them 10 or 15 years later. Hormone replacement therapy is one way to turn down the heat. So is exercise. In a study of Swedish women, those who exercised regularly were half as likely to have hot flashes as those who didn't. Because hot flashes often disrupt sleep, exercise may also lead to better, more refreshing sleep and less fatigue. Exercise's potential for coping with stress and improving mood also comes in handy during this time. In the University of Pittsburgh's Healthy Women Study, for example, women going through menopause who had the greatest increases in activity over the three-year study reported the smallest increases in symptoms of depression and stress.

Exercise for Postmenopausal Women

Many older women fear that exercise is dangerous to the heart, bones, and joints, and that what they really need to do is *take it easy.* Just the opposite is true. Older women and men actually need to be *more* active than they were in middle age. Not only is old age the period during which chronic diseases such as heart disease, cancer, and diabetes manifest themselves, but declining hormone levels make it increasingly easy to lose muscle and add fat. During this extended stage of life, regular physical activity can help:

- Increase aerobic capacity
- Maintain muscle mass
- Prevent weight gain
- Decrease the risk of heart disease
- Decrease the risk of type 2 diabetes
- Maintain bone density and strength
- Maintain joint strength, flexibility, and mobility
- Maintain cognitive function
- Maintain a positive outlook

RECOMMENDATION

After menopause, the triad of moderate aerobic activity, strength training, and stretching becomes increasingly important. Even women who were inactive through adolescence, early adulthood, and middle age can benefit from starting an exercise program late in life that includes at least 30 minutes of moderate, weight-bearing exercise such as walking each day, two to three sessions of strength-training exercises that work the body's major muscle groups each week, and regular stretching exercises.

As estrogen levels decline following menopause, you lose one of your most important shields against heart disease. In many women, dwindling levels of estrogen are accompanied by increases in blood pressure and LDL (bad) cholesterol and decreases in HDL (good) cholesterol, all of which can nudge one toward a rendezvous with heart disease. Regular exercise, along with a "heart healthy" diet, can move you in the other direction by decreasing blood pressure and LDL levels and increasing HDL. Exercise increases the body's sensitivity to the hormone insulin, thereby providing the most potent protection possible against type 2 diabetes. It also puts enough of the right kind of stress on your bones so their bone-building activities keep pace with bone-dissolving activities.

Weight-bearing exercise, along with regular stretching and strength training, are the key components of any strategy for maintaining flexibility and preventing falls. Strength training and stretching give your muscles and joints the power and flexibility to maintain—or regain—their full range of motion. Flexibility is crucial for performing everyday tasks, such as climbing stairs and getting up from chairs or into and out of car seats, as well as recreational activities, without soreness and stiffness. It also protects your muscles from injury. Strong, flexible muscles are also excellent protection against loss of balance and falling, the most common cause of broken bones in older women.

Points to Remember

- Although it is never too late to start, establishing an exercise program in the teen and young adult years can help a young woman build a greater peak bone mass and develop healthy habits she can benefit from the rest of her life.
- Exercise during pregnancy can reduce physical discomfort and improve mood. However, a woman should consult her doctor or mid-

wife for guidelines for safe and appropriate exercise during pregnancy.

- Post-pregnancy exercise can help you restore muscle strength and flexibility, help return your body to its pre-pregnancy weight and shape, minimize fatigue, and help you to maintain a positive outlook.
- If you are nearing or passing through menopause, exercise can help you maintain muscle mass, keep your bones strong, and your joints flexible. It can also help you avoid gaining weight, or lose weight you gained through your pregnancies, and help you maintain a positive outlook. It can also help to relieve some of the symptoms associated with menopause.
- After menopause, regular exercise can help reduce your risk of developing heart disease, stroke, diabetes, osteoporosis, and some forms of cancer. It can also help you maintain cognitive function and memory, ward off depression often associated with aging, and keep you mobile well into your later years.

15

Sharing the Wealth
of Good Health

Once you discover the power of small changes in diet and exercise for yourself, we hope you will use the influence you have to help others around you make these important lifestyle changes. As a mother, daughter, partner, grandmother, sister, aunt, teacher, friend, citizen, or voter, you have a tremendous effect on—and often responsibility for—the well-being of the people in your life. To a great extent, we women can shape the nation's health, once we've taken good care of our own.

Perhaps the greatest need lies with the children and older people in our lives. Statistics show that children in the United States today are less fit than we or our parents were. They smoke more, weigh more, have higher cholesterol levels, and exercise less compared with children 30 years ago. All of these factors can lead to cardiovascular disease. At the other end of the age spectrum, as sedentary, unfit older people lose their functionality, their quality of life deteriorates. This may mean more time spent in assisted living centers and nursing homes in a debilitated physical condition and demoralized state of mind.

We end this book by offering information on fitness activities for the young and the old offered through community walking programs, affinity clubs, private fitness facilities, YWCAs/YMCAs and JCCs, park and recreation departments, and senior centers and government

260

agencies. We're certain you'll find an area of interest for just about anyone in your life—if you are creative in your approach. While we can't list every opportunity in every community, we can offer a variety of general suggestions that may whet your appetite.

Fitness and Health Trends for America's Children

Spend a few minutes at any playground and the nonstop activity might convince you that America's children are in fine physical shape. Some are, but many more aren't. Consider the following troubling statistics on the health of our children:

- **Increasing inactivity, declining fitness:** The National Children and Youth Fitness Study indicates that at least one-half of all American youths don't engage in enough physical activity to promote long-term health. Only about one third of elementary and secondary schools offer daily physical education classes, and most of these aren't likely to foster lifelong physical activity. A fitness testing program sponsored by the Chrysler Fund Amateur Athletic Union, which tracks fitness among 9.7 million youngsters between the ages of 6 and 17, shows that children are getting weaker, as well as slower in endurance running. Since 1980 there has been a 10% dropoff on scores for distance runs and an 11% decline in the proportion of youngsters who achieved at least a "satisfactory" score on the entire test.

- **Increasing overweight and obesity:** The latest National Health Examination Survey found that as many as one in five children between the ages of 6 and 17 are overweight. From 1963 to 1980 obesity increased 54% among children 6 to 11 and 39% in adolescents 12 to 17. The third National Health and Nutrition Examination Study (NHANES III—1988–1991) found that the prevalence of overweight among American adolescents age 12–19 was 20% for males and 22% for females, an increase of 6% from NHANES II (1976–1980). About 17% of Mexican American boys aged 6 to 11 are overweight—the highest percentage of any adolescent group. Among African Americans, 16% of girls aged 6 to 19 are overweight.

- **Risk factors for heart disease:** Inactive children, when compared with active children, weigh more, have higher blood pressure, and lower levels of heart-protective HDL cholesterol. Even though heart attack and stroke are rare in children, evidence suggests that the processes leading to those conditions begins in childhood. More than 25 million Americans under age 20 have high cholesterol; this condition is all too common among African-American girls of all ages.

- **Diabetes risk:** Researchers in several parts of the country have shown a surprising rise in the number of teenagers with type 2 diabetes, also called adult-onset diabetes. In one of several studies, researchers at Children's Hospital Medical Center in Cincinnati reviewed the medical records of 1,027 diabetics aged 19 and younger between 1982 and 1995. They found that cases of type 2 diabetes jumped from 4% before 1992 to 16% in 1994. These results were surprising because this form of diabetes usually develops in people age 30 and over and has been considered rare in children. However, type 2 diabetes is typically associated with obesity, which is on the rise among children.

- **Smoking and second-hand smoke:** More than 2 million adolescents between the ages of 12 and 17 smoke, and their ranks are growing by an estimated 3,000 teens *a day*. Nine million American children under age five live with at least one smoker and are exposed to second-hand smoke for virtually the entire day. Combined with inactivity, cigarette smoke poses a very serious risk to the health of young people.

Inactivity, TVs, and Computers

Why are so many American kids unfit? For starters, they spend a great deal of time watching TV and playing computer games, which are sedentary pursuits. And if this inactivity weren't bad enough, children who watch television are exposed to countless advertisements for unhealthy foods, which invariably influence their eating habits. If they eat while they watch, they begin to associate television with snacking, a practice that further contributes to weight gain.

American children spend an average of 17 hours a week watching TV, *in addition to the time they spend using video and computer games.* A 1998 study published in the *Journal of the American Medical Association* showed that children who watch several hours of television a day are more likely to be overweight than those who do not. As part of the NHANES III, 4,063 children aged 8 to 16 were interviewed and examined between 1988 and 1994. They were asked how many times a week they played or exercised enough to sweat or breathe hard—including school activities such as physical education—as well as how many hours of television they had watched on the day before the interview. The children's body composition was calculated using both a skin-fold test and a body-mass index chart.

The results: overall, 26% of the kids reported watching four hours or more of TV per day; among non-Hispanic black children, the figure was 43%. The boys and girls who watched four or more hours of television per day had the highest body fat, while the children who watched less than one hour of television had the lowest. The same study also showed that vigorous activity levels were the lowest among girls, non-Hispanic blacks, and Mexican Americans. And while boys *and* girls reported similar patterns of play and exercise between the ages of 8 and 13, activity dropped off for girls in the 14 through 16 age group. Only 65% of the girls reported vigorous activity three times a week, compared with 86% of the boys.

BOX 59

Helping Your Kids to Practice Healthy Eating

- Don't keep junk food in the house; buy fruits, raisins, nuts, and low-fat dairy products.
- Limit delivery foods and trips to fast-food restaurants.
- Cut down or ban soda; replace it with water or skim milk and moderate quantities of fruit juice.
- Offer plenty of fruits and vegetables; tell very young children these are "grow big" foods.
- Absolutely no eating in front of the TV or in the car—a habit that encourages mindless overeating (and makes a mess!).
- Be a good role model. You don't have to be perfect, but practice what you preach in terms of food choices and activity levels.

What about Weight Loss?

Your child is overweight. What are the best ways to help him or her reach a more appropriate weight?

Melinda Sothern, who directs a pediatric weight management program at Louisiana State University Medical Center and West Jefferson Medical Center, addressed that issue during a recent interview on *CBS This Morning*. First off, Sothern cautioned, don't worry about the numbers on the scale unless your pediatrician has some concerns. You're better off focusing your attention on your child's eating and activity habits. "If your child seems lethargic and eats too much, it may be a sign that he or she is headed for trouble down the road," said Sothern. "Just because they appear overweight doesn't mean they'll have a problem; babies, particularly breast-fed babies, will be chunky at age two."

Your weight can serve as a guide. If you are overweight, your child may have inherited tendencies to be overweight. If he or she snacks constantly and consistently chooses TV and computers over any physical activity, you probably need to intervene and change these habits (see Box 59).

Sothern advises parents not to impose an exercise routine on kids but to encourage them to play games that get them moving. All activity counts, and it doesn't have to be continuous. Good toys for indoor activity include soft sponge balls or any soft sports equipment, jump ropes, hula hoops, and music for dancing. As your children get older, they can graduate to outdoor toys such as swing sets, basketball, skates, and monkey bars. If you don't have a yard, take them to the playground or get them into an after-school activity or sport.

How do you get your child off the couch and away from the TV set? Set firm limits on TV watching, says Sothern. She suggests making TV the last thing your child can do when coming home from school, not the first.

Appropriate Activity for Children and Adolescents

Young people who are active tend to be both physically and emotionally healthier. But how much activity do kids need? Consider these guidelines from the National Association for Sport and Physical Education and the President's Council on Physical Fitness and Sports:

- **For elementary-school-aged children:** At least 30 to 60 minutes of age-appropriate physical activity from a variety of physical activities on all, or most, days of the week. Some of the child's daily physical activity should be in periods lasting 10 to 15 minutes or more and include a variety of activities that are moderate to vigorous in nature.
- **For adolescents:** Three or more sessions per week of activities that last 20 minutes or more at a time and require moderate to vigorous levels of exertion. Adolescents should be physically active each day, or nearly every day, as part of play, games, sports, work, transportation, recreation, physical education, or planned exercise, in family, school, and community activities.

Fond, or not-so-fond, memories of physical education classes lead many of us to believe that children get at least some activity each day at school. Not so. The Centers for Disease Control's Youth Risk Be-havior Surveillance System found that among high-school students, only 43% of ninth graders attend physical education class on a daily basis; by 11th and 12th grades, the number is a mere 19%.

Getting Kids Involved in Activity—Safely

If your child or children aren't getting exercise through their physical education classes, you'll want to supplement it if you can. Participation in physical activity and sports programs can help girls (and boys) learn to value themselves for their abilities and their skills.

"You really do learn a lot of self-esteem when you play sports," re-marked two-time Olympian Marcia Pankratz to a conference on women's health in Washington, D.C. Pankratz played on the U.S. Women's field hockey team in Seoul (1988) and in Atlanta (1996). "You gain confidence . . . you really learn coordination. You learn to understand your body, especially at a time when your body's chang-ing, and you're growing up . . . You appreciate the fact that you have strong muscles and you're not a little petite thing all the time . . . [In sports] I was able to express myself . . . to give my opinion, whether it was right or wrong or anything. I learned that to compete was okay . . . I had qualities that went beyond just being a pretty girl."

Get kids involved as soon as you can, advises Wayne Westcott, a strength-training expert who often speaks to school children about fitness. "We know from study after study that if you get them excited in middle school or junior high, they'll stay with it throughout high school. If you don't, it's hard to get them started," says Westcott. "High school kids, especially girls, get very self-conscious. I recently spoke at a wellness seminar at a high school about physical fitness and strength training. Some of the boys got involved, but the girls sat there. Their attitude was, 'You don't play sports, why do you want to get into shape?' It was too late."

If you can involve your child in some form of physical activity now—whether it is a sport or dancing or martial art—that interest may last well into adulthood. Lisa, age 29, remembers how she learned to love dance as a child, which has led to an active lifestyle throughout her life. "I wasn't actually very sports-oriented as a kid. I started playing softball when I was about six. When I got hit in the head, I made my mom take me off the team. That was it for sports. But I did start taking tap and jazz dance when I was five or six. I was very shy as a child, but I learned to like performing as part of a group. It gave me more grace, and poise and confidence. I belonged to a health club in high school. I did a little bit of weight-training, stretching, calisthenics, aerobic classes and walking. I continued dance in college. My favorite thing to do now is to take aerobics classes. I like aerobics because it's so intense, and you move your whole body. You get into it for that hour, and it's really invigorating. It gives you more energy throughout the day. And I enjoy the choreography and the music so much."

An activity menu for your child should have lots of variety and change as she or he grows. Here are some suggestions:

- Active play dates with friends, preferably outdoors where there is room to romp and roam
- School and community sports: for very young children, sport activities with limited competition that give everyone the chance to participate; for older children, or for younger children who are more competitive, sports that match their drive and interest
- Active family outings and vacations
- Children's activities sponsored by YMCAs, private fitness centers, and local park and recreation departments

INTERNET RESOURCES

Looking for ideas for individual and family fitness activities? These days, the Internet is one of the best sources for fitness events. For example, *Walking Magazine* lists a wide variety of walking events by state and by month of the year at http://www.walkingmag.com/calendar.html. The American Volkssport Association hosts scores of noncompetitive walks in the U.S. every weekend. For information call 800-830-WALK or visit the Volkssport Web site at http://www.ava.org.

The Cool Running Web site (http://www.coolrunning.com) includes a calendar of running and walking events around the country listed by date, plus a handy kid's page. The Road Runners Club of

America (http://www.rrca.org) lists running events plus a link to the Avon Women's 5k race series. The 1999 schedule, for example, listed races in 15 cities across the country. When you visit these sites, keep in mind that many running events, such as a 5k race (3.1 miles), often include a walking event that is held simultaneously. Some Web sites also post race results after major races.

If your child wants to in-line skate, you can find safe instruction by calling the International In-line Skating Association at 800-56-SKATE for a list of instructors, or view a list at http://www.iisa.org, the association's Web site.

Swimming is a great activity for all ages. For youth programs, try your local park and recreation department, YMCA/YWCA, or JCC. In addition, try http://www.healthclubs.com, to search for a swim program at a private health club near you. Some private clubs now offer both youth swim programs, which may be taught by Red Cross-certified instructors, and water therapy programs for older people, some of which are taught by instructors certified by the Arthritis Foundation. Swimmers can also find help online at http://www.swiminfo.com, which offers handy workout regimens. If you have a competitive masters swimmer under your roof, try the Web site for the United States Masters Swimming, at www.usms.org. This site has discussion forums, current record times, and databases with information about pools across the country.

If you'd rather walk or hike a trail through a state park, national park, or a park in another country, try Yahoo! at http://parks.yahoo.com, which lists parks in all three categories, plus links for other activities such as boating, camping, climbing, fishing, hiking, and mountain biking. You can also make reservations for airline flights, hotel rooms, rental cars, and for the parks themselves through this site. For information on national parks, the National Park Foundation site, http://www.nationalparks.org, also lists helpful information on these national treasures, including directions to the park and details on exhibits and films, fees, and wheelchair accessibility.

Finally, getting children involved in walking for a worthy cause has many benefits. It gives them a sense of community and awareness of the importance of service to others, all the while promoting a healthy lifestyle. Raising pledges can also give children a goal to work toward and a sense of accomplishment afterward. Visit *Walking Maga-*

zine's Web site, http://www.walkingmag.com/calendar.html, for a listing of these fund-raising fitness events.

Fitness and the Elderly

If you're a member of the so-called "sandwich generation," you have aging parents who need your attention, in addition to children who need your care. Older people benefit as much from exercise as younger people. Here are some of the ways, as we describe in more detail in Chapters 2 and 11:

- Research shows that it's never too late to start exercising. Older people who are regular walkers have better climbing capacity, higher bone mineral content, lower concentrations of blood triglycerides, and a significantly larger lung volume than nonwalkers. In addition, they also have a more positive attitude toward physical activity and a higher estimation of their own physical fitness.
- Strength training can delay many typical signs of aging. These include stiff joints, weak bones, poor muscle tone, low basal metabolism, digestive difficulties, poor circulation, slow reaction time, diminished short-term memory and cognitive function, and sleep disorders.
- Simple stretching and strength-training programs—which are readily available in most communities—can reduce falls by improving mobility and balance. Elderly women who exercise moderately have been shown to have a lower risk of hip fractures than those who do light activities or are completely sedentary.
- Strength training enables older people to complete everyday tasks with more confidence. One study showed that as older people became stronger, the speed with which they could walk 20 feet increased. That's the width of a typical city street.
- Physical activity can also improve quality of life by helping older people stave off depression that may result from loss of family, friends, and their own health. Exercising in groups has an added advantage—not only do the participants feel stronger, but they benefit psychologically from group interaction and attention from the instructor.
- Finally, physical activity can prolong life. In one long-term study,

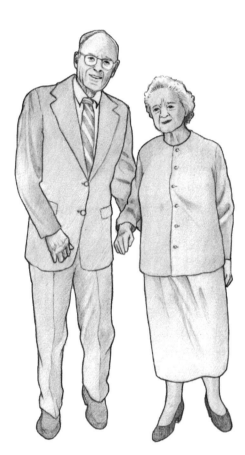

the mortality rate among the men who walked less than one mile per day was nearly twice that for men who walked more than two miles per day. These findings also indicate that walking is as beneficial for elderly people as it is as for younger individuals.

Getting Elders Involved in Activities—Safely

• **YMCA/YWCAs, JCCs:** Although services vary from location to location, YMCA/YWCAs and JCCs frequently offer training for older adults, including endurance exercises, strength exercises, water exercises, and walking. Check your local phone book for

YMCA/YWCA listings. Do the same for the JCC, or call its national headquarters at (212)532-4949. You can also visit the Web site at http://www.jcca.org.

- **Private health clubs:** Because the population in the United States is rapidly aging, many private health clubs, often in conjunction with local hospitals, have begun to offer special senior membership programs and water exercise, nutrition, and strength-training programs aimed specifically at the over 50 crowd. To find a health club in your area with such a program, call International Health, Racquet and Sportsclub Association at 800-228-4772, or visit its Web site at http://www.healthclubs.com. This site has a photo and brief description of participating clubs, as well as a search engine you can use to find a club in your area.

- **Senior centers:** Multipurpose senior centers provide recreational, social, and educational activities, as well as nutrition programs, for older people. Check your phone book for a senior center near you.

- **Departments of Aging:** These agencies, often part of city or county government, offer a wide range of resources for seniors including information on senior nutrition, rehabilitation, and recreational programs. Again, check your phone book for listings.

- **Books and magazines:** For more information on senior exercise, let us also suggest that you start with an excellent book, *Exercise: A Guide from the National Institute on Aging,* which lists the benefits of exercise for older people, self-tests, exercise that can be done at home, and important information on nutrition. You can get a free copy by calling 800-222-2225, or via the NIA's Web site at http://www.nih.gov/nia. Ask for publication NIH 98-4258.

How young can an older person be? Very young, if one well-known theatre group is any indication. Consider The Fabulous Palm Springs Follies, a troupe of singers, dancers, and comedians who play to packed houses at the Historic Plaza Theatre in Palm Springs, California. Members of the troupe, including the Legendary Line of Long Legged Lovelies, range in age from 54 to 86—some were already performing back in the days of Irving Berlin, Busby Berkeley, and Vaudeville! Don't believe it? Visit their Web site at http://www. palmspringsfollies.com and see what a lifetime of physical activity can do!

Community and Environmental Strategies to Promote Exercise

We can all play an important role in advocating for community-based changes, in our neighborhoods, schools, and workplaces, to create an environment that promotes increased physical activity.

Strategies to increase exercise should target the perceived barriers to activity. Some examples of such social, structural, and environ-

BOX 60

Community-Based Strategies for Promoting Physical Activity

Schools

- Advocate for required daily physical education for all students.
- Petition to allow school gymnasiums to be open on evenings and weekends for community recreation.
- Car-pool to provide students' transportation to and from sports practice and playing fields.

Workplace

- Advocate for employers and health care organizations to create benefit packages that include wellness programs and reimbursement for fees associated with health clubs and other recreational activities.

Neighborhoods

- Advocate for community sidewalks, walking trails, bicycling paths, safe parks with good lighting and police patrols.
- Start (or join) a neighborhood or community walking program.

mental modifications, and how we can advocate for them, are provided in Box 60. The National Association for Sport and Physical Education (NASPE) has set national standards for physical education in schools; it recommends a minimum of 30–60 minutes of daily physical activity for elementary school children and at least 45 minutes per day for middle and high school students. If your school district does not provide this, you can contact NASPE (800-213-7193) or PE4LIFE (202-776-0377) or http://www.pe4life.com for guidance.

Points to Remember

- There are a number of disturbing health trends among young children and teenagers in America. Unhealthy habits in children and teenagers, including a sedentary lifestyle, can lead to serious illness later in life. Fortunately, it is in most kids' natures to be active. Encourage them and help them to be active at a young age and they will probably continue.

- A sedentary lifestyle among the elderly can cause a loss of functionality, depression, even death. But it is never too late to start exercising, and even older, sedentary people can reap the benefits of physical activity.

- There are many health and fitness resources available for the young, the old, and anyone in between; use the Internet and your local phone book to get started.

References and Additional Resources

1. The Best Investment You'll Ever Make

Ewing, C. G. "The Benefits of Physical Activity on Coronary Heart Disease and Coronary Heart Disease Risk Factors in Women." *Women's Health Issues, Jacob's Institute on Women's Health* 7, no. 1 (1997): 17–23.

"The Health Benefits of Physical Activity." *President's Council on Physical Fitness and Sports Research Digest,* series 1, no. 1 (1993).

Manson, J. E., and I.-M. Lee. "Exercise for Women: How Much Pain for Optimal Gain?" *New England Journal of Medicine* 334 (1996): 1325–1327.

Manson, J. E., F. B. Hu, J. W. Rich-Edwards, et al. "A Prospective Study of Walking as Compared with Vigorous Exercise in the Prevention of Coronary Heart Disease in Women." *New England Journal of Medicine* 341 (1999): 650–658.

"Physical Activity and Women's Health." *President's Council on Physical Fitness and Sports Research Digest,* series 2, no. 5 (1996).

Romans, M. C. "Physical Activity and Exercise among Women." *Women's Health Issues, Jacob's Institute on Women's Health* 7, no. 1 (1997): 1–2.

Slupik, R. I., and K. C. Allison. *The American Medical Association's Complete Guide to Women's Health.* New York: Random House, 1996.

U.S. Department of Health and Human Services. *Physical Activity and Health: A Report of the Surgeon General.* Atlanta: Centers for Disease Control and Prevention, 1996.

Wiest, J., and R. M. Lyle. "Physical Activity and Exercise: A First Step to Health Promotion in Women of All Ages." *Women's Health Issues, Jacob's Institute on Women's Health* 7, no. 1 (1997): 10–16.

2. Exercise, Nature's Medicine

Bensonor, I., K. M. Rexrode, and J. E. Manson. "Physical Activity and Health in Women." In J. Rippe, ed., *Lifestyle Medicine,* pp. 343–355. Cambridge: Blackwell Press, 1999.

Carlson, K. J., S. A. Eisenstat, and T. Ziporyn. *The Harvard Guide to Women's Health.* Cambridge: Harvard University Press, 1996.

Greene, B., and O. Winfrey. *Make the Connection: Ten Steps to a Better Body and a Better Life.* New York: Hyperion, 1996.

Krauss, R. M., R. H. Eckel, B. Howard, et al. "AHA Dietary Guidelines Revision 2000: A Statement for Healthcare Professionals from the Nutrition Committee of the American Heart Association." *Circulation* 102 (2000): 2284–2299.

Mahle Lutter, J., and L. Jaffe. *The Bodywise Woman.* Champaign, IL: Human Kinetics, 1996.

Manson J. E., F. B. Hu, J. W. Rich-Edwards, et al. "A Prospective Study of Walking as Compared with Vigorous Exercise in the Prevention of Coronary Heart Disease in Women." *New England Journal of Medicine* 341 (1999): 650–658.

Manson, J. E., P. M. Ridker, J. M. Gaziano, and C. H. Hennekens. *Prevention of Myocardial Infarction.* New York: Oxford University Press, 1996.

Manson, J. E., H. Tosteson, P. M. Ridker, et al. "The Primary Prevention of Myocardial Infarction." *New England Journal of Medicine* 326 (1992): 1406–1416.

Nelson, M. E., and S. Wernick. *Strong Women Stay Young.* New York: Bantam Books, 1997.

Pate, R. R., M. Pratt, S. N. Blair, et al. "Physical Activity and Public Health: A Recommendation from the Centers for Disease Control and Prevention and the American College of Sports Medicine," *JAMA* 273, no. 5 (1995): 402–407.

"Physical Activity and Cardiovascular Health." *NIH Consensus Statement* 13, no. 3 (1995): 1–33.

Rich-Edwards, J. W., J. E. Manson, C. H. Hennekens, and J. E. Buring. "The Primary Prevention of Coronary Heart Disease in Women." *New England Journal of Medicine* 332 (1995): 1758–1766.

3. Four Steps to a New Exercise Habit: An Overview

Annesi, J. J. *Enhancing Exercise Motivation: A Guide to Increasing Fitness Center Member Retention.* Los Angeles: Leisure Publications, Inc., 1996.

Bouchard, C., and R. J. Shephard. *Physical Activity, Fitness, and Health: International Proceedings and Consensus Statement,* Champaign, IL: Human Kinetics, 1994.

Dishman, R. K. "Exercise Adherence." In R. N. Singer, M. Murphey, and L. K. Tennant, eds., *Handbook of Research on Sport Psychology,* pp. 779–798. New York: Macmillan, 1993.

———"Overview." In R. K. Dishman, ed., *Exercise Adherence: Its Impact on Public Health,* pp. 1–9. Champaign, IL: Human Kinetics, 1988.

Gauvin, L., and W. J. Rejeski. "The Exercise-Induced Feeling Inventory: Development and Initial Validation." *Journal of Sport and Exercise Psychology* 15 (1999): 403–423.

Kau, M. L., and J. Fischer. "Self-Modification of Exercise Behavior." *Journal of Behavior Therapy and Experimental Psychiatry* 5 (1974): 213–214.

Keefe, F. J., and J. A. Blumenthal. "The Life Fitness Program: A Behavioral Approach to Making Exercise a Habit." *Journal of Behavior Therapy and Experimental Psychiatry* 11 (1980): 31–34.

Leith, L. M., and A. H. Taylor. "Behavior Modification and Exercise Adherence: A Literature Review." *Journal of Sport Behavior* 15 (1992): 60–74.

"Physical Activity and Intrinsic Motivation." *President's Council on Physical Fitness and Sports Research Digest,* series 1, no. 2, (1993).

Prochaska, J. O., and B. H. Marcus. "The Transtheoretical Model: Applications to Exercise." In R. K. Dishman, ed., *Advances in Exercise Adherence,* pp. 161–180. Champaign, IL: Human Kinetics, 1994.

Sallis, J. F. "Summary of the Workshop 'Behavior Change Principles.'" *Homeostasis* 37, no. 4 (1996).

Sallis, J. F., and M. F. Hovell. *Determinants of Exercise Behavior.* Exercise and Sport Sciences Reviews 18. Baltimore: Williams and Wilkins, 1990.

4. Step 1: Plan Your Active Lifestyle

American Heart Association. *Fitting in Fitness: Hundreds of Simple Ways to Put More Physical Activity into Your Life.* New York: Times Books, 1997.

Annesi, J. J. "Effects of Group Promotion on Cohesion and Exercise Adherence." *Perceptual and Motor Skills* 87 (1999): 723–730.

Blair, S. N. *Living with Exercise: Improving Your Health through Moderate Physical Activity.* Dallas: American Health Publishing Company, 1991.

Paffenbarger, R. S., and E. Olsen. *LifeFit: An Effective Exercise Program for Optimal Health and Longer Life.* Champaign, IL: Human Kinetics, 1996.

Sallis, J. F., M. F. Hovell, C. R. Hofstetter, et al. "Distance between Homes and Exercise Facilities Related to Frequency of Exercise among San Diego Residents." *Public Heath Reports* 105, no. 2 (1990): 179–185.

"A Walking Event Tip Sheet." Insert to *Walking Magazine,* from the Editors of *Walking Magazine,* 1997.

Westcott, W. *Strength Fitness: Physiological Principles and Training Techniques.* Madison: Brown and Benchmark, 1995.

5. Step 2: Proceed with Your Exercise Program

American Heart Association. *The Healthy Heart Walking Book: A Complete Program for a Lifetime of Fitness.* New York: Macmillan, 1995.

Rippe, J. M., and P. Amend. *The Exercise Exchange Program: The Flexible Fitness Plan that Allows You to Design a New Workout Every Day for a Lifetime of Good Health.* New York: Simon and Schuster, 1992.

6. Step 3: Record Your Progress

Sallis, J. F. "Influences on Physical Activity of Children, Adolescents, and Adults." *Physical Activity and Fitness Digest, President's Council on Physical Fitness and Sports,* March 15, 1994.

Sallis, J. F., M. F. Hovell, C. R. Hofstetter, and E. Barrington. "Explanation of Vigorous Physical Activity during Two Years Using Social Learning Variables." *Social Science and Medicine* 34, no. 1 (1992): 25–32.

7. Step 4: Reward Your Efforts

Annesi, J. J. "Teaching Tenacity." *Fitness Management* 13, no. 10 (1997): 27–30, 39–40.

Belisle, M., E. Roskies, and J. M. Levesque. "Improving Adherence to Physical Activity." *Health Psychology* 6 (1987): 159–172.

Orstein, R., and D. Sobel. *Healthy Pleasures.* Reading, MA: Addison-Wesley Publishing Company, 1989.

Sallis, J. F., M. F. Hovell, C. R. Hofstetter, et al. "Lifetime History of Relapse from Exercise." *Addictive Behaviors* 15 (1990): 573–579.

10. Eating Your Way to Good Health

American Heart Association. "Dietary Guidelines for Healthy American Adults: A Statement for Health Professionals from the Nutrition Committee." *Circulation* 94 (1996): 1795–1800.

Clark, N. *Nancy Clark's Sports Nutrition Guidebook.* 2nd ed. Champaign, IL: Human Kinetics, 1997.

Finn, S. C. *The American Dietetic Association Guide to Women's Nutrition for Healthy Living.* New York: Perigee Books, 1997.

"The Food Guide Pyramid: Your Guide to Food Variety." http://www.Eatright.org/fgp.html.

U.S. Department of Agriculture. "Updated Dietary Guidelines for Americans." http://www.hhs.gov/cgi-bin/waisgate?WAISdocID=348086425+3+0+0andWAISaction=retrieve.

"X-FACTOR (Excessive Fat and Consumption Trends in Obesity Risk)." *Shape Up America!* http://www2.shapeup.org/sua/surveys/x-factor.html.

11. The Scientific Case for Physical Activity

Bensenor, I., K. M. Rexrode, and J. E. Manson. "Physical Activity and Health in Women." In J. Rippe, ed., *Lifestyle Medicine*, pp. 343–355. Cambridge: Blackwell Press, 1999.

Blair, S. N., et al. "Physical Fitness and All-Cause Mortality: A Prospective Study of Men and Women." *JAMA* 262 (1989): 2395–2401.

Gregg, E. W., et al. "Physical Activity and Osteoporotic Fracture Risk in Older Women: Study of Osteoporotic Fractures Research Group. *Annals of Internal Medicine* 129 (1998): 81–88.

Hu, F. B., R. Sigal, J. W. Rich-Edwards, et al. "Walking as Compared with Vigorous Exertion in the Prevention of Type 2 Diabetes Mellitus in Women." *JAMA* 282 (1999): 1433–1439.

Hu, F. B., M. J. Stampfer, G. A. Colditz, et al. "Physical Activity and Risk of Stroke in Women." *JAMA* 283 (2000): 2961–2967.

Kannel, W. B., and P. Sorlie. "Some Health Benefits of Physical Activity: The Framingham Study." *Archives of Internal Medicine,* 139 (1979): 857–861.

Kushi, L. H., R. M. Fee, A. R. Folsom, et al. "Physical Activity and Mortality in Postmenopausal Women." *JAMA* 277 (1997): 1287–1292.

Manson J. E., F. B. Hu, J. W. Rich-Edwards, et al. "A Prospective Study of Walking as Compared with Vigorous Exercise in the Prevention of Coronary Heart Disease in Women." *New England Journal of Medicine* 341 (1999): 650–658.

Manson, J. E., E. B. Rimm, M. J. Stampfer, et al. "A Prospective Study of Physical Activity and Incidence of Noninsulin-Dependent Diabetes Mellitus in Women." *Lancet* 338 (1991): 774–778.

Paffenbarger, R. S., R. T. Hyde, A. L. Wing, et al. "The Association of Changes in Physical Activity Level and Other Lifestyle Characteristics with Mortality among Men." *New England Journal of Medicine* 325 (1993): 538–545.

Rockhill, B., W. C. Willett, D. J. Hunter, et al. "Physical Activity and Breast Cancer Risk in a Cohort of Young Women." *Journal of the National Cancer Institute* 90 (1998): 1155–1160.

Rockhill, B., W. C. Willett, D. J. Hunter, et al. "A Prospective Study of Recreational Physical Activity and Breast Cancer Risk." *Archives of Internal Medicine* 159, no. 19 (1999): 2290–2296.

U.S. Department of Health and Human Services. *Physical Activity and Health: A Report of the Surgeon General.* Atlanta: Centers for Disease Control and Prevention, 1996.

12. Exercise for Women with Chronic Health Conditions

American Diabetes Association. "Diabetes Mellitus and Exercise." *Diabetes Care* 22, suppl. 1 (1999): S49–55.

American Heart Association. "Guide to Primary Prevention of Cardiovascular

Diseases: A Statement for Healthcare Professionals from the Task Force on Risk Reduction." *Circulation* 95 (1997): 2329–2331.

Cardiac Rehabilitation. Rockville, MD: U.S. Department of Health and Human Services, Agency for Health Care Policy and Research, 1995.

Corcoran, C., and S. Grinspoon. "Treatments for Wasting in Patients with the Acquired Immunodeficiency Syndrome." *New England Journal of Medicine* 340 (1999): 1740–1750.

National Osteoporosis Foundation. *Physician's Guide to Prevention and Treatment of Osteoporosis.* Washington, DC: National Osteoporosis Foundation, 1998.

"Physical Activity and Cancer." President's Council on Physical Fitness and Sports. *Physical Activity and Fitness Research Digest,* series 2, no. 2 (1995).

"Physical Activity and Fitness for Persons with Disabilities." President's Council on Physical Fitness and Sports. *Physical Activity and Fitness Research Digest,* series 3, no. 5 (1999).

"Physical Activity and Osteoporosis." President's Council on Physical Fitness and Sports. *Physical Activity and Fitness Research Digest,* series 2, no. 3 (1995).

"Physical Activity in the Prevention of Type II (Non-Insulin Dependent) Diabetes." President's Council on Physical Fitness and Sports. *Physical Activity and Fitness Research Digest,* series 2, no. 10 (1997).

"Physical Activity in the Prevention and Management of Coronary Heart Disease." President's Council on Physical Fitness and Sports. *Physical Activity and Fitness Research Digest,* series 2, no. 1 (1995).

Pinto, B. M., and N. C. Maryuma. "Exercise in the Rehabilitation of Breast Cancer Survivors." *Psychooncology* 8 (1999): 191–206.

"The Sixth Report of the Joint National Committee on Prevention, Detection, Evaluation, and Treatment of High Blood Pressure." *Archives of Internal Medicine* 157 (1997): 2413–2446.

13. Working the Body, Healing the Mind

Annesi, J. J. "Effects of Minimal Exercise and Cognitive-Behavior Modification on Adherence, Emotional Change, and Physical Change in Obese Women." *Perceptual and Motor Skills* 91 (2000): 332–336.

Annesi, J. J., and S. Dacey. "Muscle, Mood and Behavior." *Fitness Management* 15, no. 2 (1999): 40–43.

Carlson, K. J., S. E. Eisenstat, and T. Ziporyn. *The Women's Concise Guide to Emotional Well-Being.* Cambridge: Harvard University Press, 1997.

"The Influence of Exercise on Mental Health." *President's Council on Physical Fitness and Sports Research Digest,* series 2, no. 12 (1997).

"NIH New Advisory Statement on First Federal Obesity Guidelines, National Heart, Lung, and Blood Institute." Press Release, June 3, 1998, http://www.nih.gov/news/pr/jun98/nhlbi-03.htm.

"Special Report: The *Psychology Today* 1997 Body Image Survey Results." *Psychology Today* 30, no. 1 (1997).

14. Fitness at Each Stage of Your Life

American College of Sports Medicine. *American College of Sports Medicine's Guidelines for Exercise Testing and Prescription.* 5th ed. Baltimore: Williams and Wilkins, 1995.

Carlson, K. J., S. E. Eisenstadt, and T. Ziporyn. *The Women's Concise Guide to a Healthier Heart.* Cambridge: Harvard University Press, 1997.

National Center for Health Statistics. *National Health and Nutrition Examination Survey (NHANES), 1988 to 1994.* Atlanta: Centers for Disease Control and Prevention.

15. Sharing the Wealth of Good Health

"Adolescence: A 'Risk Factor' for Physical Activity." President's Council on Physical Fitness and Sports. *Physical Activity and Fitness Research Digest,* series 3, no. 6 (1999).

"Co-anchor Thai Assuras Gets Tips on Helping to Keep Your Child Trim, from Melinda Sothern, Louisiana State University Medical Center and West Jefferson Medical Center." *CBS This Morning.* Transcript, November 9, 1998.

"Health Benefits of Physical Activity during Childhood and Adolescence." President's Council on Physical Fitness and Sports. *Physical Activity and Fitness Research Digest,* series 2, no. 4 (1995).

"Influences on Physical Activity of Children, Adolescents, and Adults or Determinants of Active Living." President's Council on Physical Fitness and Sports. *Physical Activity and Research Digest,* series 1, no. 7 (1994).

"Physical Activity and Aging: Implications for Health and Quality of Life in Older Persons." President's Council on Physical Fitness and Sports. *Physical Activity and Fitness Research Digest,* series 3, no. 4 (1998).

"Physical Activity for Young People." President's Council on Physical Fitness and Sports. *Physical Activity and Fitness Research Digest,* series 3, no. 3 (1998).

"Physical Activity Promotion and School Physical Education." President's Council on Physical Fitness and Sports. *Physical Activity and Fitness Research Digest,* series 3, no. 7 (1999).

National Institutes of Health. *Exercise: A Guide from the National Institute on Aging.* Publication #NIH 98–4258 (http://www.cdc.gov/nchswww.releases/95facts/95sheets/fs-ad263.htm).

U.S. Department of Health and Human Services. *CDC's Guidelines for School and Community Programs.* Atlanta: Centers for Disease Control and Prevention, 1997.

Acknowledgments

Our understanding of the health benefits of exercise has been advanced not only by talented scientists but by the dedicated women and men who volunteer their time and energy as participants in research studies. The frontiers of medical science have been greatly extended by their commitment and altruism. In particular, we thank the participants in the Nurses' Health Study, the Physicians' Health Study, and the Women's Health Study for their long-term and ongoing commitment to prevention research at Brigham and Women's Hospital; we add to this our appreciation for the hundreds of thousands of participants in other research studies throughout the United States and worldwide.

This book would not have been possible without the dedication of our colleagues and the inspiration of our patients, who have provided support and encouragement for this effort. The day-to-day struggles of our patients and colleagues in adopting and maintaining a physically active lifestyle, and the desire to share the strategies of those who have triumphed, served as an early stimulus for this project. We particularly thank the women who took time out of their overcrowded schedules to share with us their experiences; their testimonials help to make this book pragmatic and "real-life."

We would also like to thank James Annesi and Wayne Westcott for providing such valuable information on exercise adherence and strength training, respectively. Fatima Valeras adapted the strength-training programs and Michael Wood the stretching program in Chapter 8; we are grateful to both of them. Sue Keller did a magnificent job creating the illustrations. Michael Wood also consulted with us on the illustrations and adapted the cardiovascular programs for the home exercise equipment in Chapter 9. Dr. Annesi reviewed the entire manuscript, as did John McCarthy, executive director of the International Health, Sportsclub, and Fitness Association. We are also particularly indebted to Patrick J. Skerrett for his invaluable contributions to this manuscript and his exceptionally insightful and sage advice.

We are also deeply grateful to our talented editors, Susan Wallace Boehmer and Michael Fisher, and the dedicated staff at Harvard University Press for their able direction, expert input, and unwavering support in bringing this effort to fruition. Evan Marshall, literary agent, also provided a tremendous amount of guidance and support.

Finally, and above all, we thank our families for their tireless devotion, support, patience, and inspiration throughout this endeavor.

JoAnn Manson
Patricia Amend

Index